Rs 320/-

HIV/AIDS and Traditional Medicine
A Journey to Dialogue

Other Books of Interest

Adaptation Biology and Medicine
Volume 1: Subcellular Basis (81-7319-11-5)
   B.K. Sharma et al

Volume 2: Molecular Basis (81-7319-246-4)
   K.B. Pandolf, N. Takeda and P.K. Singal

Volume 3: New Frontiers (81-7319-422-X)
   J. Moravec, N. Takeda and P.K. Singal

Brain Protection and Neural Trauma (81-7319-261-8)
   V.K. Khosla et al

Diarrhoeal Diseases (81-7319-343-6)
   N.K. Ganguly and N. Appaji Rao

Essentials of Clinical Toxicology (81-7319-219-7)
   S.B. Lall

Immunomodulation (81-7319-118-2)
   Shakti N Upadhyay

Immunopharmacology (81-7319-241-3)
   Shakti N. Upadhyay

An Introduction to Immunology (81-7319-334-7)
   C. Vaman Rao

Introduction to Rational Use of Drugs (81-7319-156-5)
   R.R. Chaudhury and C.D. Tripathi

Medical Diagnostic Techniques and Procedures (81-7319-350-9)
   Megha Singh et al

Multi-Drug Resistance in Emerging and Re-emerging Diseases (81-7319-346-0)
   R.C. Mahajan and Amu Therwath

Pharmacology and Therapeutics in the New Millennium (81-7319-380-0)
   S.K. Gupta

Reproductive Immunology (81-7319-262-6)
   Satish K. Gupta

HIV/AIDS and Traditional Medicine
A Journey to Dialogue

EDITOR
Ranjit Roy Chaudhury

Narosa Publishing House
New Delhi   Chennai   Mumbai   Kolkata

Dr. Ranjit Roy Chaudhury
President, Delhi Society for Promotion of Rational use of Drugs
Co-ordinator, India-WHO Programme in Essential Drugs
National Institute of Immunology
New Delhi-110 067, India

Copyright © 2002 Narosa Publishing House

NAROSA PUBLISHING HOUSE

22 Daryaganj, Delhi Medical Association Road, New Delhi 110 002
35–36 Greams Road, Thousand Lights, Chennai 600 006
306 Shiv Centre, D.B.C. Sector 17, K.U. Bazar P.O., Navi Mumbai 400 705
2F–2G Shivam Chambers, 53 Syed Amir Ali Avenue, Kolkata 700 019

All rights reserved. No part of this publication may be reproduced, stored in
a retrieval system, or transmitted in any form or by any means, electronic, mechanical,
photocopying, recording or otherwise, without the prior written permission of the publisher.

All export rights for this book vest exclusively with Narosa Publishing House.
Unauthorised export is a violation of Copyright Law and is subject to legal action.

ISBN 81-7319-471-8

Published by N.K. Mehra for Narosa Publishing House, 22 Daryaganj,
Delhi Medical Association Road, New Delhi 110 002 and printed at
Replika Press, Pvt. Ltd., Delhi 110 040 (India).

Dedicated to the memory of
Professor V. Ramalingaswami
Who left us on 28 May, 2001

Preface

This book contains the proceedings of a meeting on 'HIV/AIDS and Traditional Medicine - A Journey to Dialogue' held at New Delhi on 9th and 10th November, 2000 at which, for the first time, experts in traditional systems of medicine, researchers and clinicians in allopathy, health administrators, policy makers and media representatives discussed together the role of the traditional systems of medicine in HIV/AIDS.

There is growing interest today, both in the developing and the developed countries in the enhanced use of traditional systems of medicine for prevention and cure of disease. In the field of HIV/AIDS successful herbal treatments in traditional systems for HIV/AIDS have been reported from different parts of the world. These need to be followed up by carrying out well controlled clinical trials within the scientific framework of modern clinical pharmacology yet not destroying the concepts of the traditional system. It is hoped that the proceedings of the meeting described in this book will help towards this endeavour.

Work being carried out by Ayurvedic and other experts were presented and discussed in an atmosphere of scientific spirit of sharing by persons from different systems and different disciplines. Constraints and problems were freely discussed, names of plants used were exchanged and the group presented a series of suggestions and recommendations for future collaborative work.

We are happy to report that some of the recommendations have already been followed. An All India Network of interested persons has been set up and a protocol for clinical evaluation of traditional medicines in HIV/AIDS has been prepared. This has been published in the Journal of Alternative and Complementary Medicine (2001), Volume 7, Number 5, 2001, pp. 553-566.

We would like to thank Dr. (Mrs.) Mandakini Roy Chaudhury and Mrs. Chitra Khandelwal for help in editing the manuscript and Ms. A. Banerji and Mr. Subhash Khanna for their administrative and managerial support in organizing the Dialogue. We also would like to acknowledge our appreciation and gratitude for help and support received from Dr. Palitha Abeykoon, Dr. Jai Narain, Dr. N.K. Ganguly, Dr. K. Srinivasan and Mrs. Shailaja Chandra. We would also like to thank all the participants for their cooperation and for accepting to write up their presentations promptly so that this book could be published.

The meeting was organized jointly by the Delhi Society for Promotion of Rational Use of Drugs and the Global Initiative for Traditional Systems of Health, Oxford, and the Commonwealth Working Group for Traditional and Complementary Health Systems. It was made possible by support from the South East Asia Region Office of the World Health Organization, New Delhi, the Indian Council of Medical Research, the Population Foundation of India, UNAIDS office, New Delhi and the Department of the Indian Systems of Medicine, Government of India. We are grateful to these organizations for the help received from them.

Dr. G. Bodeker
Chairman
Global Initiative for Traditional
Systems of Health,
Oxford

Professor Ranjit Roy Chaudhury
President
Delhi Society for Promotion of
Rational Use of Drugs,
New Delhi

Abbreviations

ADCT	Antibody-Dependent Cytoxidase
AIDS	Acquired Immune Deficiency Syndrome
CDC	Communicable Diseases Centre for Disease Control and Prevention
CNS	Central Nervous System
DSPRUD	Delhi Society for Promotion of Rational Use of Drugs
FCSW	Female Commercial Sex Worker
GIFTS	Global Initiative for Traditional Systems of Health
HIV	Human Immunodeficiency Virus
ICMR	Indian Council of Medical Research
IEC	Information, Education and Communication
INH	Isonicotinic Acid Hydrazide
IPR	Intellectual Property Rights
ISM	Indian Systems of Medicine
FITC	Fluorescent Isothiocyanate
KABP	Knowledge, Attitudes, Behaviours and Practices
NACO	National AIDS Control Organization
NARI	National AIDS Research Institute
NGO	Non-Governmental Organization
NICD	National Institute of Communicable Diseases
NII	National Institute of Immunology
NRTI	Nucleoside Reverse Transciptase Inhibitors
RITAM	Research Initiative on Traditional Antimalarial Methods
RTI	Reproductive Tract Infection
STD	Sexually Transmitted Disease
UNAIDS	Joint United Nations Programme on HIV/AIDS
VCT	Voluntary Counselling and Testing
WHO	World Health Organization

Contents

Preface		*vii*
Abbreviations		*ix*

1. Introduction   1
2. HIV/AIDS: Global Scenario and the African Experience   9
   G. Bodekar
3. HIV/AIDS: The Indian Experience   14
   Q. B. Saxena
4. Problems in Evaluation of Traditional Medicine in AIDS   17
   S.A. Dahanukar
5. Clinical Trials of Two Herbal Combination Preparations on HIV/AIDS Patients: A Double-blind Study   21
   S. Rohatgi
6. The Efficacy of an Ayurvedic Drug Formulation Against HIV/AIDS   25
   R. Kuttan
7. Treatment of HIV/AIDS Patients by Ayurvedic Principles and Possibilities   29
   C.N. Deivanayagam
8. Role of Ayurveda in the Management of AIDS   32
   Suresh Chaturvedi
9. Scope of Ayurveda (Traditional Medicine) in the Management of Human Immunodeficiency Virus (HIV/AIDS): An Introduction   35
   V.N. Pandey
10. Studies on Plants for Control of HIV/AIDS in Ayurveda   42
    Shriram Sharma
11. HIV/AIDS and Ayurveda: Some Leads   44
    H.S. Palep
12. Biospermicides-cum-Microbiocides and HIV/AIDS   46
    G.P. Talwar

13. Immunomodulation as a Strategy for Restoration of
    Immunocompetence for Protection Against
    Opportunistic Infections   49
    Shakti N. Upadhyay

14. HIV/AIDS and the Use of Condoms   53
    Shashi Kant

15. An Overview of the Proceedings   57
    G. Bodekar

16. Discussion   61
    Jai P. Narain

17. Homoeopathy Trials in Patients with HIV/AIDS   62
    V.P. Singh

18. Closing Remarks   66
    Ranjit Roy Chaudhury

19. Closing Remarks   67
    V. Ramalingaswami

20. Recommendations   69

    Sanskrit Terms Used in the Text   74

    List of Contributors   75

Introduction

Professor R. Roy Chaudhury, President, Delhi Society for Promotion of Rational Use of Drugs, welcomed the delegates, invitees and participants to the two-day meeting: HIV/AIDS and Traditional Medicine—A Journey to Dialogue.

Professor R. Roy Chaudhury

The idea for a meeting on HIV/AIDS and traditional medicine was enthusiastically received and part funded by WHO. The ICMR readily agreed to participate and support it. The Population Foundation of India also extended a grant. UNAIDS promised to meet the expenses of publication of the proceedings. The Dialogue has been organized by DSPRUD and the Global Initiative for Traditional Systems of Medicine, Oxford. The press release for the Dialogue received a very enthusiastic response. At least 60 persons had called, and wanted to share their findings and demonstrate their cures as well as discuss their results. Another meeting would soon have to follow.

Dr G. Bodeker, Chairperson, Global Initiative for Traditional Systems of Health and Chairperson, Commonwealth Working Group on Traditional and Complementary Health Systems

More than 300 million people are estimated to be infected with HIV/AIDS in Africa. The Durban Conference has made it amply clear that most of them will not be able to afford modern medicines. Sick people seek healthcare. If they cannot source expensive antiretroviral medicines, they turn to traditional medicines.

An alarming forecast indicates that, in a decade or so, the incidence of HIV/AIDS in India might overtake that in Africa. Therefore, the role of traditional sector becomes extremely important in India as well.

The traditional healers in Africa have come together, collaborated with NGOs and initiated clinical trials, clinical observations and research. Their programmes are far from perfect, but they need to be commended, and not criticized, on taking the first step. The emerging trend is that there are immunomodulators which strengthen the immune system. There are instances where patients have been able to gain weight, get off their sick beds, be free of opportunistic infections and start earning for their families and greatly extend their life span. Several points emerge from the experience gained so far, but a complete picture is by no means available. The poor will seek traditional medicines for HIV-related diseases. Therefore, the traditional sector must be prepared to provide an appropriate response.

The support from traditional medicine can include appropriate medicines as also restraint on claims of cure. It can mean appropriate training in terms of identifying HIV-related illnesses, referral and traditionally acceptable methods of counselling people who are traumatized by the discovery of their HIV-positive status. It can also mean proper evidence-based evaluation of traditional medicines that appear to have a positive effect on antiviral cells as immunostimulants for HIV-related diseases. Although no attention has been paid to this area so far, their significance is being rapidly recognized in Africa.

India has more than 600,000 traditional medicine practitioners, thus providing a vast infrastructure for spreading an AIDS prevention message. A coordinated response from this sector is required. If this sector is informed about the disease, it can make a useful contribution. However, this response has to be based on a partnership with conventional medicine.

In Uganda and Senegal, the number of HIV/AIDS cases has reduced, and one of the most important reasons for this, at least in Uganda, is the multisectoral approach for tackling HIV/AIDS. This provides a prominent place for traditional medicine practitioners who have welcomed training, appreciated the evaluation of their medicines. Indeed, some of their medicines have been found to be good alternatives to expensive modern medicines.

Dr Palitha Abeykoon, Director, Health Technology and Pharmaceuticals, WHO SEARO, New Delhi

On behalf of WHO, Dr Abeykoon thanked the organizers for presenting him an opportunity to participate in this significant landmark in the efforts to meet some of the challenges the world faces as regards HIV/AIDS. He said that WHO would provide all kinds of support.

HIV/AIDS was first recognized in 1981 and has proved to be a devastating condition, as it affects the most productive segment of the population. Much can be done that is tangible or specific, but scientists are unsure about how these will work, because the variables currently involved in matters of prevention, containment and control depend on factors that are not easy to control. Two issues have emerged, namely the role of traditional medicines on the one hand, and the possibility of bringing the knowledge and heritage of traditional medicines and its practitioners to bear on this, on the other. The latter has acquired great urgency.

WHO has set up targets—very specific ones—for the control of HIV/AIDS. The first target is to reduce HIV infection by 25% among young people by the year 2005; the second is to reduce global infection by 25% by the year 2010. For the past few years WHO has been active in trying to integrate traditional medicines into national healthcare systems, a gradual process already at work in many countries. India has a great potential to offer to the rest of this region some means of bringing the best of traditional medicines and trying to integrate it with the healthcare systems. This region, and possibly the entire world, looks towards India to lead in sharing its know-how and to enable a successful culmination of WHO's efforts.

Thirdly, WHO believes that there is a need to develop "national and regional global information network exchanges" where people can share their experiences. In the SEARO region a monograph is being developed on the current status of traditional medicines. The sheer numerical strength of traditional practitioners make them a singular resource that can be tapped to deliver healthcare to every part of India. Since the early 1980s, WHO has been looking into traditional medicines and the involvement of traditional medicine practitioners in the prevention and control of AIDS, specifically in Africa.

How can the cooperation of traditional medicine practitioners be enlisted for activities such as health education, epidemiological studies, contact tracing, and even for condom promotion and distribution? How can the educational structure be revamped and adopted to prepare these practitioners to effectively participate in national activities in order to prevent and contain the spread of HIV/AIDS? The rich and vast biodiversity of India, the well-trained scientific community and the resources available both among the public and corporate sectors hold the promise for unimaginable, unprecedented breakthroughs in this area, and these must all be tapped. There is recorded scientific evidence based on a number of *in vitro* studies that some medicinal plants have demonstrated clear inhibitory effect on various aspects of HIV. Nasthonostheme, derived from the Australian chestnut tree, and *Glycerrhiza glabra* have also shown good results in the treatment of HIV/AIDS. There is immense potential with the biodiversity that is available in India. In fact, it is unlimited, if one goes about it in the correct way. There is a need to invest sufficient energy, effort and resources in this particular area to come up with something that would really help not just India but the world as a whole.

Dr G. Satyavati, Former Director General, ICMR, New Delhi
HIV/AIDS has, given the awakening call for many fields, not only for medicine but also research in basic sciences, because HIV has revealed how the body's defence system can totally break down and lead to disaster. The concept of a psychoneuron–immunoendocrine axis, which has now gained acceptance in the past 20–25 years, was already known in Ayurveda.

Ayurveda recognizes the importance of immunity, the body's host defence system in life, not just for diseases. Defence is required against any agent which induces stress, ageing or degeneration. *Ojas* is such a concept in Ayurveda. The reduction or the deficiency of *ojas* is the main reason why there is immune system failure in conditions like HIV/AIDS. Considering the claims of successful drugs against AIDS from the point of view of experts in traditional medicine, it is seen that these experts may not be talking about the anti-HIV/AIDS function of these drugs, but rather about how these medicines may improve the immune system. The same package may help in AIDS, in cancer and other autoimmune disorders. The *Rasayana* group of drugs can be used for many ailments. *Triphala, Terminalia chebula, Embelica officinale,* asparagus and herbominerals are *rasayana* drugs. These drugs must be used even when the chemotherapeutic approach is being adopted. These two approaches must be integrated in an ongoing clinical trial. The design may be difficult but it is not impossible to achieve this kind of integration. Today, all over the world modern medicine and modern science is talking about such an integration of the body and mind. Centuries ago, Ayurveda described health as *Samadosh*. It is the fourth dimension, the spiritual dimension that has been added by Ayurveda and now WHO has also included this dimension.

Certain very strong combinations of herbominerals are available, such as those used by practitioners of Siddha and Ayurveda. Western practitioners may consider these combinations as toxic, but that is the case only when the medicine is not prepared properly. If it is judiciously followed up in a scientific and rational manner, there is a strong case for using herbominerals in HIV/AIDS. Many people live with HIV infection but they do not develop AIDS, this is because of *ojas*. Thus, *ojas* should and can be promoted in many ways.

Dr Vasantha Muthuswamy, Deputy Director General and Chief (BMS), ICMR, New Delhi

Professor Ramalingaswami started the current programme in traditional medicine in the 1980s and Dr Satyawati spearheaded various aspects of the programme, which are being acclaimed nationally and internationally. *Rasayana* as a special group has been identified and the *rasayana* drugs have also been identified. The ICMR has all the plants which have to be tested and used in this research. When the very first HIV case was reported from Chennai, Professor Ramalingaswami organized a meeting; an extensive literature survey was undertaken and experts were called. Following this, surveillance centres were set up in India, and thus the National AIDS Control Organization (NACO) was created. The National Research Institute was set up to carry out intensive work in this area. ICMR examines all the claims that come to its notice regarding traditional medicines and HIV/AIDS.

Eighty per cent of those living in Africa as well as those in developed countries resort to some kind of alternative systems of medicine. Alternative systems vary from naturopathy to Chinese medicine, but most systems use plant-based drugs. There are positive effects and evidences of these cures and the moral responsibility of health professionals to examine these claims to see whether the entire mass of suffering humanity can be benefited. The rich heritage of India must be explored and the gains provided to the masses.

ICMR will see that the national heritage is preserved and propagated and brought forth for the use of the general population.

Traditional medicine is locally accessible, culturally relevant and there is historical evidence of its effectiveness in various areas. However, documentation is poor. Lack of standardization of the formulations has been the bane of this group of drugs. There are concerns of safety and an absence of regulatory mechanisms. There is a lack of common interest, trust and action, which is a significant impediment in identifying effective indigenous approaches to the prevention and cure of AIDS. Scores of medicinal plants, which may be potentially effective remain unknown and uninvestigated.

If all the foregoing issues are resolved, India can become a leader in this area.

Vaidya Shriram Sharma, President, Mittal Ayurvedic College, Mumbai

Ayurveda is the science of life, which has a wealth of information on maintaining a perfect life (*ayu*). The main plan of Ayurveda is to keep a healthy individual in perfect health. However, if the individual does become ill due to some wrong practices then Ayurveda also elaborates on how to be cured of illness without any adverse effects. Ayurvedic literature does mention medicines, but to prescribe drugs is not the main principle. Ayurveda advocates the *Rasayana* group of drugs for staying healthy and disease-free.

The current attitude of turning to Ayurveda only when the best modern medicine is inaccessible or unaffordable, as a lesser option, is not fair. Ayurveda is not the second best, it is a parallel system, just as significant, and should be accorded an equal status with modern medicine.

Since the last 10–12 months, the Government of Gujarat has established two centres for the treatment of AIDS using Ayurvedic principles. One centre is in Surat, and the other in Jamnagar; in both these places the faculties of the medical colleges are working in tandem with our *vaidyas*. First the diagnosis is made by doctors using their own criteria, laboratory investigations, etc., then the patient is sent to the *vaidyas* who use their own judgement and dispense medicines. When the patient returns at regular intervals of 8–15 days, both the experts carry out an examination and keep a record of the symptoms; however, the treatment given is according to Ayurvedic principles. The experience so far is very encouraging. Ninety-nine per cent of the patients are continuing treatment and claim they are feeling better. Patients with advanced symptoms are not included in the study.

In HIV/AIDS patients, Ayurvedic medicines must be used at different levels and those *vaidyas* who are interested and knowledgeable should hold discussions with allopathic experts before drawing conclusions.

One such medicine is the *brahmarasayana* of Charaka, which strengthens the immune system. Should this drug be found useful, it will bring relief not just to patients in India but to all.

Practitioners of the Indian systems of medicine are prepared to cooperate with allopathic doctors, but will work according to their principles and within their limitations. In this way, India will make progress and have something good to offer to the world.

Mrs Shailaja Chandra, Secretary, Department of Indian Systems of Medicine and Homoeopathy, New Delhi

The Department of Indian Systems of Medicine (ISM) pledges its wholehearted support to this endeavour. This department has a full-time commitment towards the propagation and development of six systems of medicine with Ayurveda as the largest among them.

The government has decided, for the first time, that MBBS students must be given exposure to the concepts and applications of Ayurveda, Unani, Siddha, Yoga, etc. They will not be allowed to practise these disciplines, it may not even be a compulsory examination paper for them. Modules on these systems are ready with a promise that they will soon be incorporated. Despite all the conquests that medical science has made, there is no help for people who live in the tiny hamlets and blocks in India. It is high time that the 600,000 registered practitioners be used for several public health concerns, not merely because such people cannot be given allopathic care, but because they can be offered healthcare for common ailments as well as chronic diseases for which these systems have a strength far beyond that offered by allopathy. The areas where these alternative systems are of help are the immunomodulators, *rasayana*, old age, body building, etc.

The present meeting is an acknowledgement that there is a need to use the services of traditional medicine practitioners. An essential drugs list was brought out for 319 conditions and 19 areas in which they fall, with 22,000 dispensaries in the country being asked to use them. Homoeopathy has the ability to address the psychological and psychiatric manifestations of individuals and families affected by AIDS.

The approach of this department has been to pick the best of the research already done, distil it and give it back. Recently, a meeting was held between eminent researchers and *vaidyas* of the Banaras Hindu University and other places. Seven areas have been identified and clinical trials would follow. AIDS and homeopathy have also been covered in this.

The six most important traditional drugs are *tulasi (Ocimum sanctum), nimba (Azadirachta indica), guduchi (Tinospora cordifolia), amalaki (Emblica officinalis), bala (Sida cordifolia)* and *pippali (Piper longum).* The Cabinet has very recently granted approval to the setting up of a Medicinal Plant Board. The Ministry of Education has promised to include the Ayurvedic and healthy living approach in textbooks for school children. The Ministry of Culture intends to put traditional medicines on their map everywhere, to revive interest in the ancient systems of medicine. In consultation with a *vaidya*, the Sports Authority of India had tried a long list of Ayurvedic preparations for building up endurance, stamina, vigour and vitality and they were able to show improvement in all the determinants. An expert checked if the drugs were the right choice and whether the combinations were right and standardization was properly observed, and he was fully satisfied. These same factors are relevant for the control of HIV/AIDS and would improve the sense of well-being.

The workshop in Hong Kong was on the research methodology for traditional medicines. The research at Surat should be extended to many more centres.

Dr Harsh Vardhan, Former Health Minister (Government of NCT of Delhi), Delhi

Five young people between the ages of 10 and 24 years get infected every minute, 7000 in a day; this means that 33 million are already infected, and 12 million have so far died. For people living in this part of the world, it is important to note that the geographical epicentre of the disease has shifted in the 1990s to Asia from Africa, the Caribbean and Latin America, where it used to be in the 1980s. A large majority of women transmit the disease to their children. The Indian systems of medicine and the traditional medicines may have a major role to play if health for all is to be provided. Health for all by 2000 has not yet been accomplished. In a WHO seminar in Kobe (Japan), it was unanimously resolved that alternative and Indian systems will have to be integrated to provide answers to most of the problems facing India.

On the one hand, extensive research is going on to find out new vaccines and new drugs, but there are economy-related limitations. Even if the world can develop good drugs and vaccines, would these drugs/vaccines be accessible to those in India? It is hoped that this forum will provide answers to such queries.

The Indian systems of medicine have rich traditional values: Ayurveda, as *vaidya* Shriramji has said, is not only medicine, it is prevention, culture, ethics and value. Like the relationship between husband and wife, it is of a complementary nature, together making a single unit. A large number of young Indians need advice. A perfect and thorough integration of both the health systems and the system of education has to be ensured. If, with a small input, millions of teachers and children can assuredly carry the message of positive health dissemination, the output would be tremendous.

Professor V. Ramalingaswami, National Research Professor, New Delhi
In Surat and Jamnagar, modern medicine and Ayurvedic/traditional medicine are practised side by side with the same objectives and goals, objective evaluation, and a dedication to work for mankind's benefit. The ancient systems of medicine are a precious gift to humanity. Pandit Nehru came all the way to Jamnagar to inaugurate the Institute.

It is important to tackle HIV in married women, and, as a result, paediatric AIDS because of vertical transmission. Women are already at the very end of the scale of things in India. The number of married women who are becoming

HIV-positive with every passing year, is frightening. There is an urgent need to specially address the question about how to diminish this fatal, terrible affliction among married women.

Counselling and confidential testing are important though daunting tasks. The entire system of traditional medicine is being examined in totality and not simply to find one golden nugget buried somewhere as modern medical history has shown. Much of modern medical therapy is based on substances that have been in practice in one culture or another in traditional medicine. The future will not be very different from the past in spite of our advances in genetics, molecular biology and chemistry and other fields. Mahatma Gandhiji said, "I am less worried, if so many people die because there is no cure, than your showing me a path by which others can be prevented from getting this disease."

The whole spectrum of activity should start with the promotion of health, with prevention of disease and the maintenance of health. In India, the window of opportunity for containing AIDS is becoming ever narrower, and will soon close. Here is a great opportunity to see that small epidemics do not grow into big ones. This is something that should not be allowed to happen. There are four states in northern India where the frequency of AIDS is still low. The Indian health minister has informed that the incidence of AIDS is growing in Bihar over the past 2 years. Earlier, it was asked why AIDS is so infrequent in Bihar and UP? Is it a question of insufficient reporting or is it something else?

Large areas of India are still free of HIV/AIDS. It is possible to keep these areas free of AIDS through special efforts. Poor countries such as Uganda are managing to stay free of AIDS. Senegal, and Thailand have done a remarkable job. These countries are demonstrating that it is possible to reduce transmission, and to contain small outbreaks. They are using traditional methods for doing this through public health systems. India could learn from such countries that are poor but are still doing something to handle this situation. The point is that India is still taking this disease too lightly. It is disturbing to know that in Thailand, the allocation of funds for AIDS is being reduced. Despite this, Thailand is doing marvellously and nothing should happen to change the course of its success story. Finally, there is a need to unleash a total war on AIDS, and a wonderful weapon for it in India would be traditional medicine in combination with modern medicine and molecular biology.

Dr J. S. Bapna, Director, Institute of Human Behaviour and Allied Sciences, Delhi, proposed a vote of thanks.

The indicators for quality of life are being discussed from the point of view of form of treatment, whether it is the use of medicine, psychology or of other systems. The greatest challenge is providing evidence of the efficacy of traditional medicine and correlating it with the outcome—the quality of life.

HIV/AIDS: Global Scenario and the African Experience

G. Bodekar

Although a global perspective on HIV has been documented, no such documentation is available on HIV and the use of traditional medicine. It is therefore difficult to present an overview.

In July 2000, China and Thailand collectively held a meeting on traditional medicine and HIV/AIDS and malaria. China is now openly discussing HIV/AIDS.

In October 1999, UNAIDS met at Kuala Lumpur and several papers on traditional and alternative medicine and HIV/AIDS were read. Most of them related to experimental research and primarily studied the antiviral and immunostimulant effects.

In Europe and the United States, around 80% of patients with HIV/AIDS use alternative medicine. The National Institutes of Health found that out of all the patients selected for randomized, double-blind clinical trials of a western drug, 40–60% were using complementary medicines without informing the investigators. All these were large-scale conventional drug trials and not specifically for HIV/AIDS. The patients were asked if they were taking any other type of medicine initially. The aim of this dialogue was to present a social research agenda in the field of traditional medicine. The present meeting will document a pattern of healthcare and its implementation. So the focus is not only on the pharmacological effects of a new medicine, but also on other medicines people take. First, what are the widely used alternative medicines and which of them offer the maximum benefit? Knowing this, a selection could be made as to which treatment deserves evaluation. At present, there is no rationale for evaluation. There should be a systematic approach to evaluating treatment for HIV. Social research can provide some guidance in this field. A consumer survey should be conducted to scrutinize patterns of self-medication. People continue to use medicines their grandmothers had given them or follow their family tradition. A survey of practitioners should be carried out by a social scientist before the clinical pharmacology of these drugs can be assessed. By surveying practitioners, fraternities actively engaged in this field should develop their own mobilization programmes to gather opinions and generate discussions. Similar in-house debates should be held on Unani, Siddha and other fraternities. A three-dimensional axis—high use, high benefit and self-imposed high priority medicines—would be the beginning of a structural approach for selecting treatments in traditional medicine to be evaluated. The experts owe this to the public.

Research on clinical observation is the next phase. For example, if in that matrix there are 20 different medicines which seem to have antiretroviral, immunomodulatory anti-HIV related effects either on vertical or horizontal transmission, the first stage is not to experiment with them in a laboratory. Instead, it could be regarded as naturally occurring. WHO has sound protocols to investigate this natural occurrence. It is a perfectly valid means of investigating, refining and generating a hypothesis. In this way, clinical observation is the second step in developing the research agenda.

Under the Indian Law, if a treatment is in customary use for years, it is possible to proceed to Phase III clinical trials, given adequate toxicology studies (6-week rat model LD_{50}). This is accepted by WHO and reduces a huge chunk of the conventional drug discovery route. Pharmacological research proceed alongside and does not have to precede clinical evaluation. Research and development should be linked to the public health agenda and must be accorded priority, because the crisis looming large is serious. Research is not really a part of a justifiable defensible strategy. Many countries have identified four broad areas for conducting research. First, the immunostimulator modulator area; second, HIV-related illnesses; and third, the area of viral load because the approach should be people- and public health-centred.

In the natural product area, a scientist starts looking for antiviral effects. This is a perfectly valid approach; however, it does not provide a lead. Modern medicine has not yet come up with a sufficiently powerful antiretroviral agent that would combat this deadly virus. In such a situation, the burden of proof and bulk of research in this area rests with traditional medicine. Traditional medicine actually belongs to the public health aspect of immunity in tackling illnesses.

Rethinking is required in the important area of mother-to-child transmission. As a community, doctors, health professionals and traditional medicine practitioners all need to be tolerant towards one another and work in collaboration. If the data are not perfect, the clinical effects may be striking. When presented in the first instance, studies would be necessarily less than perfect, but this paves the way to improve methodology. The present meeting is moving towards a common framework and a structured community. Two initiatives have been launched at the international levels: one on malaria—RITAM (the research initiative on traditional antimalarial methods) and the second on HIV/AIDS—research initiative on traditional healthcare. In each of these, the idea is to bring together scientists from around the world into a virtual community. Through this a consensus can be arrived at on priorities, research strategies, standard operating procedures, and to attract funding in order to organize research programmes and then move ahead with the Rapid

Response Research for this crisis. RITAM was inaugurated in late 1999, but already a community of over 200 scientists and traditional practitioners have participated and a database of over 360 published studies of traditional medicine on malaria made available. Ways to work out systematic reviews of these studies and preparations for their publication are ongoing. Clinical studies on antimalarials are ongoing, preclinical and toxicological evaluations are being made. Each disease imposes different specifications on evaluating traditional medicine and this exercise needs to be done. There cannot be a generic traditional medicine framework that will work with all diseases. Such medicines can be used as a starting point but each has to be tailored. In a short space of time, this has been done in partnership with the WHO Tropical Diseases Research Programme and it has turned out to be a successful partnership.

There already exist communities of cardiologists, oncologists, etc. There is also a community of traditional health practitioners and scientists in specific diseases. The malaria group comprises 260 plus members and is growing every week, and now the fruits of their efforts are emerging. In less than a year, the first clinical trial is under way in Madagascar and more are coming up.

With regard to AIDS, a consensus meeting was held in Nigeria in December 2000, which linked AIDS and malaria in terms of priority to develop a set of research methodologies in order to evaluate traditional medicine for HIV/AIDS.

The generic issue of supply and demand of the medicinal plant is known; what is to be realized is that certain diseases can drive demand. Agricultural scientists and conservation committees all have to be part of the AIDS network that is being established in India. Once a particular medicine is known to be efficacious, there would be a sudden rush and companies would not necessarily be ethical or sustainable in their practices which could lead to a depletion of stocks.

The African potato in South Africa, Zambia, Swaziland and Mozambique, is high in sterols and sterolins; it stimulates CD4 production. It is widely used in Africa by people who are HIV-positive and have full-blown AIDS. It is being developed by a South African company into a drug, but the intellectual property challengers claim that this was pirated from traditional practitioners without consent or a benefit-sharing contract. All the issues of traditional medicine practitioners are packed into this case: sustainability, intellectual property rights, and related issues. An integrated programme will look into all these issues.

At the Kenya Medical Research Institute, researchers are looking at anti-HIV activity *in vitro*. They have already identified 10 plants that have this effect. Their aim is not to produce actual ingredients and put them through the conventional drug development route, but to simply produce herbal treatments that are sound and standardized and can be used by the community.

In Uganda, an NGO—Feta Traditional and Modern Health Practitioners together against AIDS—plays a coordinating role between research and efficacy. This requires them to chair a task force that has been set up in partnership with UNAIDS to bring together research groups and NGOs in order to examine the use of traditional medicine in HIV/AIDS. They are committed to rapid research response to important treatments and have already conducted research on herpes zoster. They have evaluated Ugandan herbal treatments for HIV-related diarrhoea and have found it to be highly effective. They also found that people could gain weight up to 30 kg with simple herbal treatment in about 6 months.

Much research is being carried out in western Kenya as well. Fifty per cent of hospital beds are reserved for HIV-related illnesses. Another group in Tanzania (Tanga AIDS) are looking at thrush and have developed a very successful antifungal drug.

Dr Darshan Shanker's foundation has been working to produce herbal medicines, which is a very practical approach, given the research framework, standardization and collection.

At the Mulebeli College of Medicine in Dar es-Salaam, Tanzania, scientists are looking for antiviral agents. They are evaluating traditional medicines which show increase in CD4 and CD8 counts. They are also examining plants which appear to treat minimal levels of viral load.

It is very expensive to carry out viral load assessment which costs Rs 5000 per test. This is too expensive for people involved in traditional medicine, yet it is extremely important. Two different sources—a medical school and the Pasteur Institute—reported that there are no detectable levels of viral load in over 100 samples from Zambia and Togo. It is also not known if this indicates a cure. It is also not known whether or not the viral load increases when the patients are taken off the drug. There is a need to set up a national service for viral load detection. The National Institutes of Health, Bethesda is willing to help set up one or two centres in each region for viral load assessment in patients using traditional medicines.

In Nairobi, scientists are studying the *neem* (*Azadirachta indica*) tree. The Swahili word for *neem* is "tree that cures forty diseases". They use *neem* for malaria as a preventive and curative medicine. At the Nairobi University, they have found that *neem* also has an antiviral effect.

There are challenges in developing a research strategy for HIV/AIDS in traditional medicine. Unless there is a research infrastructure, false claims will proliferate. When traditional medicine practitioners give a certain medicine to an HIV patient and the patient feels better, they claim it as a cure. But the person is not cured. He is still HIV-positive, hence education and training is of paramount importance. A regulatory framework is necessary. In Ghana and Zambia, traditional medicine practitioners have set up their own regulatory systems. In Zambia, all the traditional medicine practitioners have set up a "Traditional medicine police". They go and apprehend wherever they find false claims being made. In Africa, the police are frightened of traditional medicine practitioners; believing that these practitioners have some secret powers. So self-regulation is very important.

In Africa, practitioners want and welcome training. In South Africa, 1500 traditional medicine practitioners were trained and almost a million people were treated. The same is true for Mozambique. The training has to be peer-based, i.e. by one traditional medicine practitioner to another traditional medicine practitioner in an acceptable language. This was done successfully in Brazil. There was a significant change in the prejudicial attitude towards transmission of HIV in people who were trained. There was a far greater knowledge about identification of HIV/AIDS symptoms.

The gender dimension is also important. Ninety-five per cent of women in antenatal care, who only had their respective husbands as their sexual partners are testing positive for HIV in Mumbai. In Africa, many *dais* (midwives) want to stop practising. Seventy per cent of the births in Africa are by traditional birth attendants. Who is going to do this work if they stop working? Infant and maternal mortality will rise. The *dais* are afraid of contaminated blood so kitchen gloves were provided to them from time to time instead of expensive sterile surgical gloves; protective aprons were also used.

In Ethiopia, women are growing medicinal plants for HIV/AIDS as a micro-industry.

Political will is of paramount importance in this area. In Nigeria, the government substantially increased the budget for evaluation of claimed cures. This is needed in India as well. The President of Nigeria is the head of the council evaluating the claims in traditional medicine in HIV/AIDS and malaria.

A list of antiviral and immunomodulatory drugs is currently available in India.

Scientists, traditional medical practitioners and people living with HIV/AIDS must be part of the research partnership, so too the NGO community and public sector, among others.

HIV/AIDS: The Indian Experience

Q.B. Saxena

Traditional medicine has always been a part of Indian homes and of every individual's growing process. It promotes self-cure.

ICMR had initiated, at the instance of Professor V. Ramalingaswami, former Director- General, ICMR, surveillance even before any HIV/AIDS case was detected. Based on referral and surveillance centre inputs, the first case of AIDS was detected in 1986. The risk behaviour of AIDS was identified, its prevalence projected, its increase quantified and a national control programme was formulated. This resulted in the establishment of the National AIDS Control Organization (NACO) by the Ministry of Health and Family Welfare in 1992.

It was now time to go into basic research and operational research. National agencies such as NARI were set up in 1992. These are carrying out extensive research into various fields of epidemiology, immunology, clinical pathology, virology, molecular biology, etc., through extramural projects at NARI and some other centres.

Through NACO it is believed that there are 94,451 HIV-positive cases and 13,304 cases of AIDS. There is a high prevalence of HIV only in some Indian states. Maharashtra, Tamil Nadu and the northeastern states have a higher prevalence. In Calcutta there are risk factors but no prevalence of HIV-positive cases. In Patna there is HIV/AIDS, but reporting is incomplete. Is it a fault of the reporting system or do Indians have some protection against AIDS that others do not have?

Some 30–35% commercial sex workers are known to be affected, except in Calcutta. Of the sexually transmitted disease (STD) cases that come to Mumbai and Pune, about 25–30% are affected; 3–4% of antenatal cases are also affected, which is very high. NARI has a cohort, which is followed up in sexually transmitted disease (STD) clinics. The surveillance by NARI showed that 9.5% males are HIV-positive, 20–22% per year for female sex workers and 6.5% in married monogamous women. The married women are infected by their respective husbands about whose conduct they are not aware. This is a serious matter.

It is important to establish the prevalence of subtypes for HIV infection in India. We have found a recombinant between A and C in the same individual.

HIV C subtype is most predominant; CT genotype is similar to the South African strain and homologous to the Zambian prototype strain as well. In the northeastern region of India, transmission is mainly due to intravenous drug abuse and the prevalence has gone up to more than 80%. This came as a surprise. There is a high risk of seroconversion in female sex workers.

Allopathic medicine is currently being used only in limited cases. There is no national policy on HIV treatment. Pilot studies are in progress and it will be some time before the outcome is known, especially for studies on vertical transmission. Treatment is being given in private hospitals and clinics and the disease is managed for opportunistic infections by standard treatment.

Very few rigorous clinical trials have been conducted in traditional medicine for HIV-positive cases. Very little data are available for clinical studies in the western style. Researchers are thus unable to use these data to carry out further clinical studies.

People are taking traditional medicine for symptomatic treatment of the illness, they may also be taking it without any illness to maintain health. Traditional medicine is believed to generally boost the immune system. It is used to treat opportunistic infections, neoplasms, etc. It is also used to obtain relief from the side-effects of conventional retroviral drugs. Canadian and American studies have revealed that people in these countries also take traditional medicine.

ICMR receives several claims regarding the effects of traditional medicine. There are very few review articles in journals. Many plants are available in nature that possess anti-HIV properties. Not all plants can be used; some may be toxic. A large control study has never been carried out and reliable data are missing. Scientists are looking for evidence to go on to Phase III trials. There is ample government support, and funding is available. Systematic studies, systematic observations, and compilation of existing data are required.

Traditional medicine practitioners are skeptical about western medicine. This impedes the evaluation, formulation and development of a public health programme. Though there are various claims, these have to be proved scientifically.

A certain conditioning is required for alternative medicine. There are effective drugs but no vaccine is available. Drugs that are available are expensive and it is not known which drugs work effectively in India, as nobody has carried out any pilot trials. Thus, understanding alternative medicine could be one of the ways.

In 1993, clinical protocol guidelines, drafted by Professor R. Roy Chaudhury and a group of experts at Chennai, were developed on how to screen a product. The person claiming a cure had to provide a biodata and mention his/her clinical experience plus the availability of an infrastructure. This not only requires finances but coordination with allopathic medicine, so that the claim can be scientifically verified. A clinical protocol for testing was developed which needs to be updated. The estimation of viral load could also be included in this programme.

The Indian population has different CD4 values as compared to the American population. The CD ratio is also different, CD values are lower and the CD4 cell count is lower. These values need to be modified in the follow-up protocol as well.

There are many reports of antiviral substances such as *Glycyrrhiza* in alternative medicine. NARI has facilities for testing any antiretroviral drug in alternative medicine. Some antiretroviral ingredients have been tested. Still, there are many unanswered questions, including standardization and bioavailability of the product, whether the product is palliative or not, is it available in plenty and, most important, whether it is cost-effective. Primarily, it needs to be known whether the medicine has any direct effect on the virus or it is merely an immunopotentiator.

Problems in Evaluation of Traditional Medicine in AIDS

Sharadini A. Dahanukar

The AIDS epidemic has stimulated an unprecedented body of biomedical research which, in turn, has led to a major expansion of knowledge in many aspects of this infection. However, researchers are still far from their goal. Despite decades of dramatic progress, AIDS remains a challenge to the physician. An important facet of HIV/AIDS everywhere is the tremendous surge of interest in the role of traditional systems of medicine in offering valid therapeutic alternatives. In spite of spending millions of rupees on this exercise not much has been achieved. One of the major reasons for this state of affairs is the multiplicity of problems that face clinical research in traditional therapies for HIV/AIDS.

The problems faced today in clinical research in HIV/AIDS can be broadly classified into the following:

1. Problems in correlating the disease process in traditional and western medicines
2. Evaluation of holistic versus drug therapy
3. Design of the study
4. Economics of conducting the study
5. Ethical issues

These points are considered in detail as follows:

1. The most contentious issue at hand is that Ayurveda does not describe any syndrome that can be classified as HIV/AIDS, and there is no clear-cut description of the syndrome in the ancient Ayurvedic texts.

Certain symptom complexes appear to sound similar to some of the symptoms associated with AIDS, e.g. *sannipatik jwara* (fever), *Pratiloma rajyakshma* (tuberculosis) and *ojakshaya* (immunodeficiency/general debility).

There is also mention of syndromes with symptoms similar to AIDS-related disorders, e.g. the clinical manifestations of different stages of AIDS can be correlated with various *kshaya* (deficiency) symptoms described in Ayurveda as follows:

- Full-blown AIDS—*Majja shukra ojakshaya*

Symptoms described in Ayurveda include: *bhrama, timir darshana, asthi soushirya, shukra prasek.*
- AIDS-related complex—*mamsa meda asthikshaya*
  Symptoms described in Ayurveda include *indriyadourbalya, krishangata pleehavridhi, atisaara asthipeeda.*
- Progressive generalized lymphadenopathy—*rasa raktakshaya*
  Symptoms described in Ayurveda include *angamarda, glanee, aruchi.*

Significantly, the concept of healthy carriers cannot be explained using the Ayurvedic philosophy.

All these complexes are subjective in nature and very difficult to diagnose even for an Ayurvedic physician. The terms used in the description of these complexes are very difficult to understand in relation to modern scientific knowledge, e.g. what exactly is *oja*? If this question cannot satisfactorily be answered, then it is not justifiable to say that *ojakshaya* is AIDS. It is difficult to label *ojakshaya* according to any biochemical parameter. From the research point of view, by making attempts to correlate the ancient and modern concepts of the disease, the researcher may be starting off on the wrong foot. This naturally can lead to a wrong choice of parameters which, in turn, can lead to false-negative (or -positive) results.

2. Ayurveda lays strong emphasis on the holistic approach in therapy. Thus, apart from the drugs used, other therapies such as *panchakarma* or diet therapies are also recommended. When a therapy is selected for evaluation, there is a tendency to be a reductionist and choose one herb or a combination of herbs without giving any thought to the patient as a single entity. This may vitiate results, and false-negative results may be obtained. For example, evaluation of immunomodulators or *rasayanas* of Ayurveda may not meet with the same success as perhaps a holistic syndromic approach.

Even among the available drugs, Ayurvedic principles must be borne in mind while selecting them for evaluation. Several agents may prove useful in different groups of patients, e.g. *rasayana, jeevaneeya, agnivardhak* or *shukravardhak.*

In case of AIDS, therefore, the following measures may be worth exploring:

- *Satva vardhak* diet
- *Panchakarma*
- *Snehan:* for protection of skin from opportunistic infections
- *Vamana:* for protection of the lungs and gastrointestinal system
- *Nasya*

Unfortunately, therapy with these approaches is far simpler than a scientific evaluation. Thus, while designing a clinical trial for such holistic therapies the major problem faced by a clinical pharmacologist is how to evaluate this holistic therapy—what controls to use, whether a placebo can be designed let alone used, leading to the next question, namely, what study design would be ideal?

3. In general, before designing any clinical study, the following factors need to be defined.

- Inclusion and exclusion criteria
- Parameters of assessment
- Treatment groups
- Clinical end-points

In each of these areas, the following problems arise while evaluating traditional medicines.

- AIDS is a disease with an unpredictable natural history. A patient may come with any symptom from the list of major/minor symptoms described as diagnostic criteria for AIDS. Hence, in order to include a large spectrum of patients, one may have to keep the inclusion criteria very flexible. If this is done, then it is equally important to quantity patients to facilitate.
- Another problem regarding the inclusion criteria is whether to include a patient in a study based on Ayurvedic symptomatology and examination findings or on the basis of modern investigations such as seropositivity, CD4+/CD8+ ratio and viral load.

In assigning parameters for assessment, confusion stems from the dichotomy of the two systems of medicine. If strictly modern research methods are applied to assess a traditional, holistic therapy, there must be cogent, reproducible, statistically valid parameters of assessment. The question then arises whether to use Ayurvedic symptoms or use changes in investigative parameters such as viral load or CD4+/CD8+ ratio to assess the response to therapy.

It may be worthwhile to consider the use of both. Just as a useful union between the two systems of medicine is advisable, in the same way a blend of both systems could be considered while choosing parameters for assessment. A certain weightage could be given to Ayurvedic signs and symptoms, quality of life parameters and laboratory diagnosis.

Placebo-controlled studies would be impossible for evaluating traditional therapies in AIDS, as it is unethical to leave patients without treatment after diagnosis. Therefore, evaluation of drug therapy *versus* holistic therapy is a major problem. Considering these issues, it appears that randomized controlled trials are difficult to plan in AIDS.

4. In the present scenario, maintaining a balance between ethics, high scientific cadre and international acceptance *versus* the economics of a trial is a tightrope walk. A clinical trial on AIDS throws up far more economic and ethical issues than any other trial at present. In order to solve these problems in a balanced way, a coherent research policy at the national level must be created and implemented.

In conclusion, all those symptom complexes found in Ayurveda that are similar to AIDS are described as *kashtasadhya/asadhya* (difficult to cure). A detailed and scholarly study of Ayurveda is needed to identify therapies with a high potential. Considering the problems regarding design of the study, simple/open pilot studies may be planned at first. Different formulations may be tried at different centres and the results must be centrally assessed to judge the best therapy. A network of laboratories will deliver results in the shortest possible time. More weightage should be given to Ayurvedic parameters of assessment and quality of life parameters while evaluating traditional medicines.

Finally, it is necessary to reiterate that research in AIDS as well as research into research methodology is necessary, particularly in the area of traditional medicine.

Clinical Trials of Two Herbal Combination Preparations on HIV/AIDS Patients: A Double-blind Study

S. Rohatgi

Prior to the discovery of sulfa drugs and antibiotics, the medical profession used to depend almost entirely on the immune system. Since the 1930s and 1940s, with the discovery of Sulfa drugs and penicillin, the emphasis of treatment of microbial infection became focused on the elimination of causative bacteria by these drugs. Newer antibiotics were developed when resistance to the existing ones was observed. During the course of complete dependence on antibiotics it was forgotten that the body's own defence forces, namely the immune system, simultaneously plays an indispensable role. No efforts were made to examine the effect of antibiotics on the immune system. The emergence of HIV/AIDS and the re-emergence of tuberculosis should have led the scientific community to examine the situation created by the drop in cell-mediated immunity in both the cases. The obvious step in the treatment of HIV/AIDS is to correct immunodeficiency. Western medicinal agents have many constituents that cause immunodeficiency, but none that correct it. Ayurveda offers drugs which can potentiate the immune system and therapy is based on the application of these drugs. All drugs which are developed in the West should be screened for their effects on the immune system and if found to cause immunodeficiency, should be avoided as far as possible.

There is no definite drug for curing AIDS. Hence, the present thinking is to improve the quality of life of an HIV patient and to delay the onset of AIDS. The first step is to screen all conventional drugs in use today and also new drugs being developed for diseases leading to immunodeficiencies. The second step is to avoid any drug in the treatment of AIDS which may cause immunodeficiency; these include known immunosuppressants such as corticosteriods. Even ointments such as betamethasone can cause irreversible immunosuppression. Hence, in such cases substitutes from Ayurveda and homoeopathy should be tried.

There was a patient whose CD count was 526 which dropped to 456 despite all precautions. On enquiry it was found that the patient was applying betamethasone ointment on his thighs to relieve irritation of the skin. This steroid was absorbed through the skin and caused chronic immunodeficiency, which did not respond readily to immunomodulators. The hypothalamus–pituitary–adrenocortical axis has a profound influence on the immune system. The approach that HIV/AIDS is incurable is negative and becomes a hindrance in the recovery of a patient. Once patient tested positive for HIV, he thinks he is doomed. A young man was found to be HIV-positive. This upset him and his family. He was constantly under surveillance. If he smoked a cigarette or had a glass of beer, it was considered sacrilege. His original CD4 count of 704 dropped to 512 due to depression. Efforts were made to boost his confidence and to change his mental attitude. He is reported to be better, has been lifted out of depression, and is optimistic about his future. His overall health is improving and the CD count would rise.

Treatment should be started soon after exposure, before the infection has established itself in the body. At this stage, is easier to treat the patient. A villager was told to use a condom as a safeguard. Since his CD4 count had gone up, he was worried that he would not have an answer for his wife. His parents and his wife's parents would get anxious if his wife did not conceive. Hence, using a condom was out of the question. Presently, the only thing available is a condom and its use depends entirely on the man. Many men simply refuse to use it. A large number of people go to town looking for jobs. They pick up the infection and when they return to their village, they spread the infection. It is imperative that steps be taken to prevent this from happening.

A young man was being treated for HIV/AIDS infection. Enquiry revealed that his wife was also HIV-positive and that she was pregnant. He was advised to put his wife immediately on immunopotentiators. Soon after birth, the newborn was also put on immunopotentiators in the form of drops and the mother was forbidden to breastfeed the child. The child's health is normal. The child was tested at the All India Institute of Medical Sciences, New Delhi after 3 months and found to be HIV-negative. This could be an effective method for prevention of vertical transmission of the disease.

Tuberculosis (TB) is the largest killer in the world today and problems are being encountered in its treatment. This is because multidrug-resistant TB is becoming resistant even to the latest cocktail of four drugs. Immunosuppression is caused by rifampicin and isoniazid and severe hepatotoxicity is caused by isonicotinic acid hydrazide (INH). The patients responded positively when Ayurvedic drugs were used alongside. This certainly appears to be a breakthrough.

In about 40–50 cases treated in Mumbai, it was observed that the CD4 count has come down with a simultaneous increase in the cytotoxic CD8 cells. Patients have gained weight and their general condition has improved.

CD4 cells result in a reactive oxygen intermediate, whereas the initial class I complex results in the increase of CD8 cells and the release of nitric oxide intermediate. Some researchers believe that both these processes develop in tandem, but opinion has it that only after the CD4 cells are no longer functioning, the CD8 counts come into play. The nitric acid route involves the conversion of arginine by enzymes in the presence of some trace metals, e.g. iron, copper, zinc, selenium and vitamin D3. These trace metals should be supplemented to promote the nitric oxide route and the reactions observed. The NACO should not depend entirely on WHO and other such organizations, because the average Indian just cannot afford these drugs.

The biggest impediment in the trial and control of HIV/AIDS cases is the absence of testing facilities. Manipur and Imphal in northeastern India report nearly 20% of all such cases. Anxiety is felt about the spread of the disease. It is affecting young people and drug users. This infection can be transmitted through contaminated needles. The health activists are providing fresh needles and persuading people not to share them. They have also set up rehabilitation centres. However, so far, NACO has not been able to supply the Regional Medical College in Imphal with a Western blot testing kit for CD4 and CD8 cell counts. All major towns should have testing facilities as it is not safe to transport blood to be tested 3 days later at another distant centre.

A young pregnant woman was given two units of contaminated blood. She picked up the HIV unknowingly. The delivery was normal, but the newborn started having diarrhoea which continued for 4 to 5 months. The suspicion was confirmed: mother and child tested HIV-positive. The father was HIV-negative. The Ayurvedic combination helped. All are healthy now. AIDS is basically an immunological problem. The host defence plays an important role in preventing the establishment of HIV in the system. Correction of immunodeficiency is the essential factor in eradicating the AIDS syndrome. Drugs which affect the immune system adversely are contraindicated in the treatment of AIDS. Antibiotics in general suppress the immune system. There is also a possibility that the emergence of HIV/AIDS is due to the continuous depressing effect of the present-day drugs. It is not wrong to suggest that AIDS is man-made. The imperative need is caution and discretion in the use of potent antibiotics and corticosteriods for viral and undiagnosed infections. Infections such as TB respond to the inclusion of immunomodulatory drugs in the therapy.

Potentiation of the immune system to eradicate opportunistic infection should be the key. The only way the re-emergence of infectious diseases can be explained is on the ground that the body's immune system has been compromised.

Note

Two combinations were used for the treatment of HIV/AIDS. One is Livzon which contains the following five plants:

- *Phyllanthus niruri*

- *Tinospora cordifolia*
- *Terminalia chebula*
- *Phyllanthus emblica* and, probably *triphala* (*Terminalia chebula, T. belleria, Emblica officinalis*)

This potentiates the liver and removes toxic free radicals, and thus cancer, TB (drug-resistant) and HIV patients are treated with it.

The other drug is Imminex which contains:

- *Holarrhena antidysenterica*
- *Picrorhiza kurroa*
- *Swertia chirata*

Patients are put on this drug till the CD4 count rises to 400–600. This occurs in about 6 months. The drug is then stopped. It is not known whether the CD4 counts decrease after the drug is stopped. This recipe that potentiates the immune system is given in Ayurveda and was obtained from an Ayurvedic practitioner treating cases of polio.

The Efficacy of an Ayurvedic Drug Formulation Against HIV/AIDS

R. Kuttan

The Amala Cancer Research Centre in Thrissur, Kerala, India caters to the section of people who are rejected on health grounds for entry into the Gulf countries. It works towards helping and pacifying such people. The objective of this work is to determine the immunomodulatory activity of herbal preparations used in traditional medicine and to find out their use in immunodeficiency states such as cancer, AIDS, etc. Thereafter, this work aims to develop an economically viable drug for use in HIV/AIDS under Indian conditions.

HIV affects mainly the CD4 lymphocytes, which results in immunological imbalance in the body and a weakened resistance to several opportunistic infections, eventually leading to death. The available medicines decrease the viral load and also lead to a deterioration of immunity.

Indigenous Indian medicines are known to stimulate the immune system. *Rasayanas*, which are preparations made either from a single plant or a combination of several plants, are well known for their immunomodulatory properties. The immunostimulating activity of plants such as *Tinospora cordifolia, Withania somnifera, Panax ginsing, Viscum album*, etc. have been studied in detail.

Three types of drugs have been developed.

NCA is a powder and a *jeevaneeya* drug. It maintains the *ojas* and reduces *ojas* depletion which occurs in the body due to HIV/AIDS. It is also indicated in several chronic diseases. Its composition is as follows:

Sanskrit name	*Botanical name*
Satavari	Asparagus racemosus
Gokshura	Tribulus terrestris
Musali	Curculigo orchioides
Amrita	Tinospora cordifolia
Chitraka	Plumbago zeylanica
Tila	Sesamum indicum
Sunti	Zingiber officinale

Sanskrit name	Botanical name
Maricha	Piper nigrum
Pippali	Piper longum
Bhallathaka	Semecarpus anacardium

+sugar, honey and ghee (clarified butter)

AC-2. This is also a powder. It improves and maintains the appetite. It is also an immunomodulatory and a *pachaniyum* drug that improves the metabolism.

Sanskrit name	Botanical name
Lavanga	Syzygium aromaticum
Nagakesara	Mesua ferrea
Ela	Elettaria cardamomum
Maricha	Piper nigrum
Pippali	Piper longum
Sunti	Zingiber officinale
Aswagandha	Withania somnifera
Haridra	Curcuma longa

+sugar

Withania somnifera is the main ingredient (about 50%). *Piper longum* is an immunomodulatory agent which increases the bioavailability of other drugs. *Curcuma longa* is antiviral.

SA-III is a drug that maintains body weight. It is indicated in tuberculosis and is a *Brahmanum* drug. Its composition is as follows:

Sanskrit name	Botanical name
Pippali	Piper longum
Pippalimulam	Roots of Piper longum
Chavya	Piper chaba (roots)
Raktachitraka	Plumbago rosea
Chitraka	Plumbago zeylanica
Sunti	Zingiber officinale (dried powder)
Yavaksharam	Natural K_2CO_3

+ghee, milk

Pippalimulam is an immunomodulatory drug.

These drugs are prepared at the Ayurvedic Research Centre, Thrissur. The extracts are not put into capsules as that is not the way of dispensing medicine in Ayurveda.

Semecarpus anacardium and *Plumbago zeylanica* definitely act as antiviral agents. Many of the other drugs are *rasayana* drugs. These drugs probably improve the depletion of *ojakshaya* which is present with HIV infection.

Initially, all three drugs are given to people who come to the Ayurvedic Research Centre. Once they feel better, only one drug may be continued which is usually SA-III. It is also given to HIV carriers. However, the treatment has to be continued for years to improve immunity even though there may be no symptoms. This is done to stabilize immunity in the body.

Some animal experiments were also conducted. NCV extract of five doses of 50 mg each per mouse was given to Balb/C mice. When the weights of the organs were taken, it was found that the weight of the thymus had increased by about 70%. The total WBC count, total neutrophils and lymphocytes had also increased. All these counts dropped when administration of the drug was stopped. This is probably because the immunity did not increase permanently. The drug could augment blastogenesis of the lymphocytes in mice. The number of antibody producing cells and titre had increased following treatment on the 5th and 6th days. Natural killer cell activity and antibody-dependent cytoxidose (ADCT) increased in normal mice given NCV. This indicated that the drug has some immunostimulatory activity.

About 5 to 6 HIV-positive patients come every week to the hospital and the Ayurvedic Research Centre. Some of them are carriers while some have full-blown AIDS.

When a patient comes to this Centre, the first tests to be performed are the Western blot and ELISA. The patient is then referred to the Ayurveda or homeopathy centre for treatment. The doses given are as follows:

1. NCV—5 g twice daily
2. AC-2—5 g twice daily followed by a glass of milk
3. SA-III—13 g twice daily.

Initially, all the three drugs are given to the patient. As the symptoms improve and the patient stabilizes, either AC-2 or NCV is continued.

Evaluation was carried out in 450 patients who were treated for a minimum of 6 months. The main problem was that as the patient felt better, he went off to the Gulf countries and stopped the treatment.

The patients were between 20 and 30 years of age. There were 364 males and 79 females suffering for a minimum of 6 months to 14 years; the majority of them had been suffering for 3 to 6 years. There were 210 asymptomatic carriers, 172 with AIDS-related complex, and 68 with full-blown AIDS. Only 45 cases with AIDS-related complex were evaluated.

Symptoms	Total cases	Cure
Fever	42	33
Diarrhoea	11	9
Lymphadenopathy	9	5
Ulcer on penis	4	2
Cough	17	11
Glossitis	13	4

Loss of appetite	20	13
General weakness	18	11
Joint pains	12	10
Insomnia	10	7
Tuberculosis	14	9
Itching	12	9
Anorexia	6	4
Herpes	2	2

When a patient had an additional TB infection, he/she was told to take antitubercular drugs available free of cost from other hospitals. Some infections such as oral candidiasis were treated by allopathic medicines and only then was treatment started at the Ayurvedic Research Centre. The monthly cost was Rs 108 for NCV, Rs 84 for AC-2 and Rs 124 for SA-III. So the total monthly cost for the three drugs was Rs 316 out of which Rs 158 was subsidized. If a patient is taking only one drug such as AC-2, the cost comes to Rs 84 which is subsidized to 50%.

An ICMR project was undertaken to evaluate the activity of the drugs and CD4/CD8 status of the patient if the CD4 count was below 200. The counts were estimated at Vellore Hospital following 3–6 and 9 months of treatment. There was a gradual weight gain for 6 months, but between 6 and 9 months there was no increase. This may be due to the fact that the patient had not taken the drugs or that the counts were actually deteriorating. The effect on CD3 and CD19 cells was also studied, but no conclusions could be drawn from the results. This might well be due to the late start of the treatment. CD4 and CD8 lymphocytes were also estimated but did not show much change. These patients had begun to feel better; there was an increase in their appetite, body weight as well as in their metabolic activity. The depletion of immunity was improved. Although many symptoms improved, the drug was less effective in cases of full-blown AIDS. There was no seronegativity although the drug was continued for 4 years or more. This is definitely a cheaper way to manage HIV patients.

Treatment of HIV/AIDS Patients by Ayurvedic Principles and Possibilities

C.N. Deivanayagam

Work is being carried out at the Government Hospital of Thoracic Medicine, Tambaram Sanatorium, Chennai, Tamil Nadu. This health centre has been in existence for more than 70 years. In 1992, the number of patients treated in all categories was 39,000, whereas in 1999 the recorded number of visiting patients crossed 97,000. The death rate earlier was 3.2 per hundred, which improved to 1.5, but has now risen to 1.7 because of HIV infection. It is noticed that the ratio of HIV patients vis-à-vis total hospital patients was 42% in May 2000 and 54% in November 2000. This is not a common phenomenon in India, but is true of the situation in Tambaram.

The current problem lies in the growing number of patients who seek care for TB and HIV. The hospital is fast becoming an HIV sanatorium. Patients are presenting with either a new TB infection or relapse of TB. Patients with HIV are likely to develop TB. Presently, there is no problem of multidrug-resistant (MDR)-TB in HIV. This situation is, however, at variance with the experience elsewhere in the world.

The sputum is cultured and tested at the ICMR Tuberculosis Research Centre. The experience of past 8 years has been that MDR-TB is no longer a problem. The active therapy for TB is given not only for 6 months, but is continued for more than 9 months. This is found to be highly beneficial for all the patients. Secondary prophylaxis is either with isoniazid alone or isoniazid and rifampicin. This is given to patients who have had therapy earlier, those who may have a scar, or those who come with advancing HIV disease.

There is one patient whose viral load was 8000. He was put on Siddha drugs along with drugs that control opportunistic infection, and the viral load has remained below the measurable level (fifty copies (pieces) per millilitre of plasma) for the past 10 months. This is a record. The Siddha approach (Siddha means expert) is mainly based on the use of herbs, sea products, natural minerals and metals. It has the same principles as Ayurveda and is as ancient as Ayurvěda. The drugs are manufactured by a complex system of grinding, pulverizing and heat processing. This results in elemental and chemical clinical transformation. The Siddha system defines health as the harmonious coexistence of the three humours of the body, namely *vata* (wind), *pitta* (bile) and *kapha* (phlegm).

The modern biomedical system is practised all over the world, but it has its limitations. The bonding or one-to-one relationship between the doctor and his patient has now completely changed to institutionalized care.

It should always be remembered that high technology is not necessarily high-quality care. Clinical skills involve careful and sympathetic listening, observing the body language of the patient and family, a careful and complete physical examination and assessment of the tell-tale signs. "*Tamaram* tongue" refers to a conglomeration of findings of the tongue: baldness of the tongue, hypertrophy of areas of the tongue, complete change in colour from the normal pink to magenta: sometimes pale, sometimes light grey. Addison disease can be diagnosed by looking at the palms. It is important to identify melanosis of the palms which is noticeable but doctors keep looking for the levels of steroids in the blood.

What is meant by the biomedical approach to post-HIV care? Hit hard, hit early and continuously. This is a sledge-hammer approach to the disease. It focuses on elimination of the enemy—the virus.

Instead, the focus should be on learning to live with the virus. This is where the Siddha system comes in. The approach in Siddha is to strengthen the mind and body and to carefully regulate the air that is breathed, the water that is drunk, the food that is eaten, avoidance of certain foods and regular exercise. In this system, drugs are tailor-made for each patient; alternation of the drug formulation is carried out from patient to patient. Just as no two finger-prints match fully, two patients infected with HIV may not match. Siddha drugs are not antiretroviral. They strengthen and restore harmony, and thus the immunity in the system. It is not merely immunorestoration that they achieve, it is the harmonization of the entire body system. Sixty-five per cent of patients have responded well to Siddha treatment. Their symptoms are under control. They have returned to work and have shown an improvement in their appetites.

In many patients the CD4 count has shown an increase, whereas for many the viral load has shown a decrease. However, this has not been achieved for all patients. Thirty patients were tested for viral load. Whatever the treatment, a reduction in CD4 count was recorded. In fact, a few patients achieved levels of viral load below the measurable level, the determination being conducted by the reverse transcriptase polymerase chain reaction (RT-PCR) and not by the β-DNA method.

Since 1993, double blood control and open-label studies have been carried out at the Tambaram Hospital and they have identified a staple regimen called RAN specifically for use in HIV infection and disease:

Table 1. Staple regimen (RAN)

Rasagandhi	Meshugu	500 mg b.d. (a compound preparation)
Amukkara	Chooranam	5 g b.d. (powder of *Withania somnifero aswagandha*)
Neelikkai	Lehyam	10 g o.d. (*Emblica officinalis/Amalaki* and other drugs)

The secret of kuttan is *rasagandhi,* which consists of mercury and sulfur. However, this has not been able to help in the case of advanced HIV infection as well as brain or central nervous system (CNS) infection, cryptococcal infection, or extensive TB or toxoplasmosis. Patients with these conditions die. In the past 8 years more than 8500 patients have died and many patients are dying.

More search and research for effective Siddha drugs is required, as is their comparison with antiretroviral therapy in multicentred trials. It is also necessary to combine them with antiretroviral therapy and then to compare them with antiretroviral therapy alone under precise laboratory conditions. More drugs and combinations with other physical methods (Yoga, exercise) and diet regulation need to be studied.

A multi-aim, multicentre controlled trial using modern drugs and Siddha needs to be set up to identify the long term results and asses the comparability of trial therapies.

There is an urgent need to standardize and utilize CD4 cell testing and RT-PCR, as well as to define laboratory conditions. These surrogate markers must be defined very clearly and universally used. The prognosis of HIV infection using Siddha treatment appears hopeful.

DISCUSSION

> Q. Professor R. Roy Chaudhury: Were the drugs in the regimen continued, tapered off or stopped?
> A. Dr Deivanayagam: They were continued for at least 5 years. They were initially stopped after 40 days of therapy. But then it was found that the symptoms recurred and the CD4 count kept falling, hence they are now continued. However, some patients discontinued the therapy. On return, some reported that they had continued to maintain the benefit, while others appeared to have lost it. There is no clear answer to the following question: whether one should introduce structured interruption or follow cyclic therapy. These answers can only be forthcoming from the *vaidyas*.

Role of Ayurveda in the Management of AIDS

Suresh Chaturvedi

HIV/AIDS is a new name, but it has been mentioned in Ayurveda. Infection with HIV is a global challenge for human immunity and vitality. Human life has a fourfold objective—*chaturvedapurushartha*. *Dharma* means duty, *artha* means earning money, *kama* means fulfilment of desires and *moksh* means attaining salvation. These can be achieved only if one is healthy both physically and mentally, i.e. *prasantmaindrayana indrigas* or mind and soul. Everybody has to be totally healthy and happy. Ayurveda believes that diet, sleep and sexual self-control are the keys to total fitness. Diet has to be in accordance with the Ayurvedic test that are the *vijayams*. After the digestion of food, there are *sapta* (seven) vital components—*ras, rakta* (blood), *mans, meda, asthi* (bones), *majja* (bone marrow) and *shuhresjevan*. These seven vital components are obtained on a daily basis from birth to death through diet. Hence, a healthy, controlled and regular diet is essential. Ayurveda has one more component to bring the total number of vital components to eight, namely *ashtadhatu* (*ojaṣ*). *Ojas* is the final vital component from the diet. There are eight drops of this *ojas* that help the heart in its regular functioning and vitality, i.e. providing strength and proper management of the heart. One ounce of *ojas* goes to the brain and regularizes brain activity and the remaining goes to the rest of the body. In this way, all activities can be performed properly and gracefully. Sleep is equally important to keep fit. A proper formulation of the body's metabolic vital components is necessary.

There is a third dimension, namely balanced, controlled sex. Controlled sex in Ayurveda is described as *brahmacharya*. *Brahmacharya* here means the brain; *brahamanda* refers to the brain's mental power. If sexual desires can be controlled, the semen would increase and divert the *ojas*. *Brahmacharya* is described in the Bhagavad Gita: "*Dharmavithebhishu kamoshi bharth shava*"—proper intercourse or sex is not harmful. But sex is not just intercourse in Ayurveda, which describes eight types of *maithuna*—*smaranam, kirtanam, keli, prekshnam, bhuyabhasnam, sankalp, adhyavasaya* and *kriyanravitti*. These *asthanedamaithun* cannot be explained adequately in modern terms. If the semen is discharged internally then *ojas* is reduced in the body and the result of this can be seen in an AIDS patient. However, AIDS is not transmitted only during intercourse; when *ojas* is reduced a person can get AIDS. *Ojas* stimulates the whole body, heart and brain. Depletion of *ojas* is the primary cause of AIDS and all these symptoms are described in Ayurveda.

The question that now arises is whether HIV is a viral or an infections condition. The known mode of transmission is from one person to another. This is not totally contradictory. In Ayurvedic literature, there is a mention of infectious diseases. *Prasangat, dhatusamparkat, nishswas* at *sahabhojanat, ekshaiya, sanachapia, vastramalya*, etc. are all routes of transmission. Ayurveda does not claim that AIDS is not transmitted, but that is not the only way of contracting this disease. *Kushtam, jwaram, shoshanecham* should be looked for *kshya* and *shosha* are different. A high index of suspicion is needed. *Vayu* will increase in the body. *Vayu* in nature leads to dryness so that semen or *ojas* will become dry. This is called *shosha*.

In Ayurvedic literature, when one talks about *rajakshama* or TB, two types are implied: *anuloma* and *pratiloma* from *rasadhatukshaya* and *shukradhatukshaya*. *Rajakshama* is a *shosha*. Ayurvedic saints have written a chapter on *rajsakshama* in *shosha*. *Shosha* is a condition after the *kshaya* (TB). Now even modern science accepts that HIV is a condition which follows TB. In Ayurveda it is the condition of a developed stage of *rajakshyana*. This condition develops after TB and can be transmitted from one person to another, similar to any infectious disease.

Ayurveda claims that the symptoms of *ojas shosha* and those of AIDS are almost the same and Ayurvedic clinicians also face these problems in diagnosis—*dhatukshinatav murcha* (giddiness) and memory loss. In Ayurveda, two types of symptoms are described, namely *sadhya* and *asadhya*. The following symptoms are considered to be those of *sadhya*, namely thin body, high temperature, loss of appetite, body washing away (*bharas*) and general reduction in strength. The following symptoms are described in cases of *asadhya*, where the patient becomes weak and has a bad odour. Such a patient appears to be untreatable. Is there a way to treat such patients? There are some guidelines. The cause has to be eliminated and some vital *ojas* medicines are to be administered. *Sandaxpani* provides the guidelines for Ayurvedic treatment. These medicines are commonly available in the market and are useful in the treatment of TB (*rajakshama*) as well as for AIDS patients.

Rasayanadravya preparations are available. *Dravyas* are single medicines and only one can be used in such cases. Some *siddha aushadhis, vasantamalti rajamriyanka* and *swarnpanpati* are also used. The extracts of *neem* (*Azadirachta indica*), a globally known tree, is also used. The seven parts of *neem* are used efficaciously; leaves, bark, internal bark, external bark, fruits, flowers and seeds. The gum of the *neem* is very useful for AIDS patients, though this fact is not widely known.

If *brahmarasayana, chyavanprash* or any *rasayana* drug is prescribed, it can be mixed with one or two *ratis* of fine *neem* gum powder depending on the age of the patient. Usually 2 ratis i.e. 4 grains of fine powder can be mixed with *sitophaladi churan*. According to modern science, as *neem* gum has antiviral properties, it can be used for viral conditions. Gum is the essence of *neem* just like semen is the *sar* of the vital component of a body. A small dose of *neem* gum would cause no complications, no side-effects, and it would definitely have an excellent positive effect. *Pathya* or the diet has to be prescribed to the patients as advice about precautions to be taken.

After the 1998 conference/workshop of NACO, all details and reports of cases are maintained. Fifty patients were treated—43 males and 7 females. There were two children below 20 years of age, 24 patients between 20 and 30 years, 21 patients between 30 and 40 years, and 3 patients above 40 years. Out of the 50 patients, 10 dropped out and 26 have felt relief. Patients tend to discontinue once their condition shows improvement. They go about their daily routine. Presently, there are 14 patients continuing regular treatment.

Ayurveda can be used advantageously for physical fitness, mental well-being and external pleasure, and in the face of the challenge of HIV/AIDS, it can come to the rescue of mankind.

Scope of Ayurveda (Traditional Medicine) in the Management of Human Immunodeficiency Virus (HIV/AIDS): An Introduction

V.N. Pandey

A variety of therapeutic procedures is being offered currently for many clinical disorders through the Indian system of medicine, especially Ayurveda. There are questions regarding the way these procedures function inside the human body and also about their logistics. Ayurveda is a science of the medical discipline based on the laws of nature, which throws light on various phenomena related to human existence. The theory of *loka-purushasamya* (macrocosm and microcosm continuum) suggests that an individual living being is a miniature replica of the universe as a whole. Both the individual and the universe are essentially *panchabhautika* (i.e. made up of five basic metaphysical factors or protoelements, namely *akasha* (ether/spare), *vayu* (air/motion), *teja* (fire/radiant/metabolic energy), *jala* (water/cohesive factor) and *prithvi* (earth/mass). The individual (*purusha*) and the universe (*loka*) remain in constant interaction with each other and also devise and draw strength from each other in order to achieve and maintain a state of normalcy and homeostasis. This exchange follows the law of *samanya* and *vishesha* (homologous *versus* heterologous) on the simple principle that a similar/ homologous matter increases the similar while a dissimilar/heterologous matter decreases or depletes the same. As long as this interaction is wholesome and optimum, man is in an optimum state of health but when this harmonious interaction breaks down, a disease state results. These *panchamahabhutas* have been further condensed and transformed into *triodoshas* (functional biological entities). Therefore, Ayurveda defines life as a union of the body, sense, mind and soul. Thus the living man, a man of action (*karampurush*), is a conglomeration of the three humours or *tridosha* (i.e. *vata, pitta* and *kapha*).

There are a variety of descriptions of a higher spiritual body available in the *Gita, Upanishadas* and *Maulikasiddhantas* (the fundamental principles of Ayurveda). These attributes act as the causative factors for the creation of the universe. The human body is an offshoot of this creative aspect. In recent years, the concepts of mental, astral and ethnic body have emerged. These three important aspects are being debated upon by modern thinkers, philosophers, scientists and also by modern medical investigators. Much information is available on the spiritual, astral, ethereal and mental attributes. Ayurveda puts forward the concept of *manas shareer,* which has three components—*satya, rajas* and *tamas.* At times they are equated to a psychological aspect but they do have *panchabhutika* or organic elements, hence they need to be distinguished. In treating a person, the physiological, mental, spiritual factors need to be considered and, therefore, the treatment offered is defined and designed accordingly.

In today's context, systems like *Chakras, Nadis,* Yoga, Acupuncture, Meridian, Bioenergy and Electronic are very much part of treatment procedures for the well-being of a person. They do not precisely depend on the mechanism of action as understood on the basis of physicochemical parameters, but their effects are being deduced through scientific experiments. The modern system of medicine is trying to elucidate their impact on the human body through the central nervous system, including the peripheral nervous system. Surprisingly, a recent study on DNA material has revealed that DNA decoding does not contain information on special placement of specific tissues. The presentation of factors governing differentiation does not help to explain this phenomenon. The concept of *atama* in the spiritual context cannot be brushed aside and can explain this aspect from the Ayurvedic point of view. Holographic studies have revealed that there is an element which is a form of energy and is capable of forming matter which can crystallize energy, but the converse has yet to be proved. This part is being investigated by atomic scientists with the hope that an answer will emerge. The Ayurvedic concept of *pancha tamantras* leading to the formation of *panchamahabhutas* bears resemblance to this supracosmic transformation. The same *panchamahabhuta* theory is also applicable to the entire plant kingdom which is being made use of in the management of HIV/AIDS.

Ayurvedic scholars have repeatedly emphasized that it is not always necessary to name a disease. Therefore, if the name of the disease is not known, the Ayurvedic physician should have the capacity and wisdom to identify *doshas, dushyas* and their combinations and permutations, i.e. *dosha–dushya sammurchana.* All types of diseases have a *samprapti* or phogenesis. It is well known that there is an incubation period for the full manifestation of a disease. The classical doctrine of Ayurveda refers to the six stages (*shadakriyakala*) of a disease process. These stages are *sanchaya, prakopa, prasana, asthansamshroya, vyakti* (manifestation) and *bheda* (differentiation). The physician can intervene at any of these six stages. It is also called a time for action. Nowadays, most patients are made aware that a physician needs to act in the early stages. There is also the concept of the *strotas* and *shrotoavarodha* (ultra-microchannels and impediments to their flow). All biological activities are processed, monitored and governed through these channels to maintain a balance and to keep the ongoing life process intact in a highly intricate manner. Apart from the *tridoshas*, seven basic tissues (*sapta dhatus*), i.e. *rasa* (plasma), *rakta* (blood), *mamsa* (muscles), *meda* (fat or adipose tissue), *asthi* (bone), *majja* (bone marrow) and *shukra* (*rajas* for female and *sperma* for male) are constantly engaged in maintaining the structural precision in a well-defined format. These *saptadhatus* have *prasada* (pure) and *kitta* (unusable) parts. There are three *malas* (excretions) which constitute the body matrix (*deha*).

Ayurveda as a system of medicine evolved and developed around these basic doctrines. A wide range of therapeutic measures are described in the system. These measures help in achieving the triple objectives of maintaining good health, preventing ailments and curing diseases.

The *pancha karma chikitsa* (five purificatory and detoxifying measures) and *rasayana* (means and measures to promote strength, vitality, integrity of the body matrix, enhancement of memory, intelligence, mental faculty, augmentation of general immunity, avoidance of decadence, preservation of youthfulness, lustre, complexion and voice, etc.) have received wider clinical application and popularity. These rejuvenating efforts are projected as a step towards replenishment of *rasadhatus* which are the nodal centres of metabolic activity of the body as a whole.

Ojas, or vital essence, is another important factor that needs to be mentioned; it is of two types, namely *para* and *apara*.

Search *versus* research

It is noteworthy that there is an ongoing debate among the scholars of Ayurveda about the scope and role of Ayurveda in restricting the spread of HIV infection and treatment of AIDS. The method of studying, analysing and understanding the physical phenomena is very useful in the physical domain. Objectivity stands as a hallmark in the management of these clinical disorders. All practitioners of medicine know that medicine is not a precise science, and that it can be formulated in terms of mathematical derivations. However, certain observations do find approval. The issues which are receiving utmost attention regarding the management of HIV/AIDS can be summarized as below:

1. Name of the disease
It is not necessary to name every disease and it is also not possible to have a name for all the diseases. Therefore, the Ayurvedic physicians have been advised to study the pathogenesis (*dosha, dhushya, samurchana*) of the disease and offer treatment accordingly.

2. Incubation period
Shadakriyakala. There are six appropriate occasions (*sanchaya, prokopa, prasara, asthansansarya, vyakti, bheda*) for the Ayurvedic physician to act.

3. Srotavarodh

Obstruction to micro- and macro-channels leading to the dominance of catabolic activities of the *dhatus* (*rasa*—plasma, *rakta*—blood, *mansa*—muscle, *meda*—fat/adipose tissue).

The concept of ultra-microchannels (*shrotas viman*) is unique in Ayurveda. All biological activities are processed, monitored and governed through these channels to keep life processes intact. Therefore, this system emphasizes the cleansing of these channels as being of paramount importance in medical management.

Asthi—bone, *maja*—bone marrow, *skhukra/rajas*—sperm/ovum, *ojas*—vital essence

The seven *dhatus* (essential constructs) which constitute, regulate and sustain the structural dynamics of the human body are independent. The concept of *ojas* emerges as an ultimate essential link in the lives of all human beings. It continuously adopts a downward trend in a condition of *oupsargika ojakshaya* which is a dominating factor in HIV-positive/AIDS cases. Its dwindling trend ultimately leads to a total loss and death.

4. The principles of proposed treatment

a. *Vyadhipratyaneeka chikitsa*: The measure (s), means and medicaments which help in developing in-built resistance to the disease are *dharaka, poshaka, rasayan* and *santarpaka dravyas*. A few examples follow:
   (i) *Panchakarma chikitsa* (five purificatory measures)
   (ii) *Kalpa-rasayan*—single or compound preparations which act as enhancers of the immune system (immunomodulators/immunoaugmentators).
   (iii) *Kshamala-vardhaka*—preparations which help in improving the physical and mental strength of the body.
   (iv) *Kshatipurtikar*—provision of supplements to replenish the loss of body constituents.
   (v) *Sthaneeyaprayoga*—local applications.
b. *Hetupratyaneeka chikitsa*: Preparations which can help in reducing/reversing/eradicating and stopping the proliferation/spread of virus (viron).

Recommended treatment

On the basis of the foregoing analysis, the recommendations made by individuals and different sources can be categorized in the following order:

A. Single drugs

Sanskrit name	Botanical name
1. Jivanti	Dendrobium macraei
2. Aswagandha	Withania somnifera
3. Satavari	Asparagus racemosus
4. Atmagupta	Mucuna pruriens
5. Bala	Sida cordifolia
6. Haritaki	Terminalia chebula
7. Vibhitaki	Terminalia bellerica
8. Amalaki	Emblica officinalis
9. Varuna	Crataeva nurvala
10. Sigru	Moringa pterygosperma
11. Bhoomyamalaki	Phyllanthus amarus, schum and thom Phyllanthus niruri hook f.non Linn.

B. Simple preparations
1. Pancha tikta guggulu
2. Maha manjisthadi kwat
3. Punarnawadi kwat
4. Sheeta paladi churna
5. Kanchan guggulu
6. Gandhak rasayan

C. Compound preparations
1. Swarna vasanta malti
2. Swarna malani vasanta
3. Sidha malani vasanta
4. Betal ras
5. Bajra vasma
6. Shilajatwadi lawo
7. Har gauri ras
8. Prabal pristi

At present there is no organized attempt to demonstrate the efficacy of Ayurvedic preparations in the management of HIV-infected individuals. There are instances when patients of HIV/AIDS have approached Ayurvedic physicians for treatment. Recently, an attempt has been made by the State Government of Gujarat in collaboration with the Jamnagar Ayurvedic University to offer Ayurvedic treatment to HIV-positive patients. The efforts are in the initial stage.

A clinical study entitled "Role of Ayurvedic drugs in HIV treatment: A preliminary study on HIV-positive patients" has been pursued at Pune. The following collaborators have participated in this study: Senior Advisor

(Dermatology and Venereology); Principal, Lokmanya Tilak Ayurved Mahavidyalaya; PG trainee (Dermatology and Venereology), Command Hospital (SC); Classified Specialist (Dermatology and Venereology), Command Hospital (SC); Classified Specialist (Medicine and Immunology), Command Hospital (SC), Pune.

Fifty patients with HIV infection were selected and randomized into two groups. One set of 25 patients received Ayurvedic drugs while the other 25 received placebo treatment for 3 months. Twenty-five HIV-seropositive patients were administered Ayurvedic drugs in consultation with the Lokmanya Tilak Ayurvedic Medical College, Pune. The Ayurvedic preparations consisted of *guduchi (Tinospora cordifolia* [wild] *miers, satavari (Asparagus racemosus* [wild]*), amalaki (Emblica officinalis Gaertn), bhoomya-malaki (Phyllanthus niruri), makaradhwaja, vanga bhasma, abraka bhasma*, in different combinations. In selected cases, bloodletting to the extent of 62–100 ml on two occasions at intervals of 15 days was done. Patients who lost more than 3 kg of weight a month were excluded.

After 3 months of the Ayurvedic drug trial, the patients were evaluated and a comparison with the control group revealed a statistically significant weight gain in the treated group as compared to the control group. The other laboratory parameters showed no significant differences between the study group and the controls, which may be because of the short duration of follow up (3 months). It may be pointed out that the more sensitive prognostic markers like CD4/CD8 cell count, P-14 and beta-2 microglobulin estimation were not done. The study is ongoing and keeping the foregoing possible factors in mind, and have included a large number of cases. Ayurvedic drugs will be continued for longer periods and the researchers expect to subsequently publish their findings.

The modern view

In the mid-1990s, conventional medicine adopted several new principles of treatment for HIV infection. Several new methods of rapidly measuring the effects of drugs on HIV in the blood, e.g. separation of plasma HIV and RNA levels, and an understanding of the rapid replication of HIV even in the clinically inactive stage of infection, have been introduced. This has brought about a change in the initial approach. A combination of drugs is being used which is not only sometimes harmful but also expensive. A brief summary of antiretroviral drugs is given in Table 1.

Future prospects

The future medicine of mankind will not be a monopoly of any one particular system of medicine. The paradigm of biomedicine—modern medicine—scientific medicine is under serious debate, keeping in view the future frontiers of human health and curative measures and, therefore, a shift has taken place

Table 1: Antiretroviral drugs—nucleoside reverse transcriptase inhibitors

Generic name	Abbreviation	Usual adult dose (oral)	Possible/adverse effects	FDA status as of mid-1998
Zindovudine	ZDV.AZT	300 mg b.i.d.	Anaemia and leukopenia, rarely pancreatitis	Approved
Diadanosine	ddl	200 mg b.i.d. If >60 kg; 125 mg b.i.d. if <60 kg	Peripheral neuropathy, pancreatitis	Approved
Zalcitabine	ddC	0.75 mg. t.i.d.	Peripheral neuropathy, pancreatitis	Approved
Stavudine	d4T	40 mg b.i.d. if >60 kg; 30 mg b.i.d. if <60 kg	Peripheral neuropathy rarely pancreatitis	Approved
Lamivudine	3TC	150 mg b.i.d.	Severe hypersensitivity	Approved
Abacavir	—	300 mg b.i.d.	Severe hypersensitivity	Under investigation

in the recent years. Old and new perspectives on the Ayurvedic system of healthcare are presented below:

Old	New
Primitive	Holistic
Ineffective	Cost-effective
Marginalized	Locally available
Becoming extinct	Undergoing revival, renewed reconstruction
Needs to be regulated	Needs to be promoted
Pharamaceutical industry	Economic value
Active ingredient model	Synergistic activity concepts

Since 1989, the interest in alternative medicine has surged by 60% in the developed world and the market is growing at an annual rate of 30%. Therefore, there are affirmative possibilities in the search for prevention and cure of chronic diseases, particularly HIV/AIDS.

Studies on Plants for Control of HIV/AIDS in Ayurveda

Shriram Sharma

The approach of Ayurveda is according to *ojas*, *ojakshayas* or *shoshas*, *pratilomas ksnayas*, etc. Ayurvedic centres in Gujarat prescribe a composite treatment consisting of *avaleha* or paste, decoction, tablet, etc. If some new symptom or opportunistic infection arises, certain specific drugs are used. The Surat experiment has been going on for 11 months and the Jamnagar one for 8 months. The response has been good, with 99% of the patients continuing with the medication. Patients who were continuously losing weight are no longer doing so. In a few cases, there has been a weight gain of half a kilogram to one kilogram. All the patients feel happy and confident about life.

One cannot definitely pinpoint any one plant as being the remedy for HIV; one can only say that the plant is beneficial.

Many plants have been discussed, e.g. *guduchi* (*Tinospora cordifolia*), *bala* (*Sida cordifolia*), *amalaki* (*Emblica officinalis*), and they are all useful. *Vaidyas* can make a contribution by treating patients according to Ayurvedic principles, which are known to them and are contained in the Ayurvedic texts.

In the Gujarat project, practioners of modern medicine observe and clinically examine the patients and laboratory investigations are also carried out. All parameters of modern research are used in these centres.

The research methodology of Ayurveda is laid out clearly in the texts and these parameters are used to conduct research even today. Knowledge or literature is collected, analysed, then discussed among other Ayurvedic physicians. The methodology of Ayurveda is known as *siddhi*. *Anusandhan*, or "research" is the process of trying to delve deeper into the details of the method, when very little about something is known.

Ayurvedic practitioners could work on their own lines and help modern physicians whenever required. Ayurvedic physicians working with modern physicians honour all the criteria and proformas laid down by WHO and the UN and will learn from control studies and blind or double-blind studies in clinical trials.

All the Ayurvedic drugs under discussion are very useful, either singly or in combination. During a discussion with a 91-year-old research worker in New York, the importance of *ghee* was observed. A drug was working well in the laboratory but had no effect clinically. However, the same drug yielded excellent results in the form of an oily preparation. Charaka gives a very elaborate description of *ghee*. According to him, when a drug has proved ineffective in certain conditions, it will prove efficacious if prepared with *ghee*. The same is the case with gold, which is not only a medicine in itself but also makes other medicines doubly effective if prescribed in combination. This has been investigated by the *vaidyas*.

As most *vaidyas* treat AIDS patients at a personal level, they should not be expected to adhere to all the formalities of research. Many such patients say that they have benefited from the treatment. The personalized treatment of a patient by a *vaidya* and research on the drug/drugs effective in the treatment of AIDS are two different things.

Ayurvedic physicians are open to clinical trials and research in collaboration with allopathic physicians. They are willing to accept any procedures required to be formulated in keeping with modern parameters, whether for publication or global assessment. *Vaidyas* treat patients according to their own criteria, so there is no clash of interest.

Ayurvedic physicians would probably have a lot to offer if they were allowed to try their hand at tackling AIDS.

HIV/AIDS and Ayurveda: Some Leads

H.S. Palep

Ayurveda should not be regarded as a science of antiquity. It has much to offer by way of the discovery of future medicines for HIV/AIDS. What are the leads one could take from Ayurveda?

The incidence of sexually transmitted diseases (STDs) is high in Mumbai: 40–50% in a clinic, about 64% in red light areas and 30% in general hospitals. Vertical transmission is almost 30%. The treatment for HIV infection cannot be continued lifelong as it has severe toxic manifestations. It damages the mitochondria. The cost of treatment, too, is prohibitive.

According to an old legend, there was a *Visha Kanya* who was a vivacious seductive woman, seducing the enemy king and killing him by slow poisoning. Was she transmitting HIV infection?

Charaka says that when the bone marrow (*majja*) matures, it produces sperms. Modern science holds that the red marrow in children matures to yellow marrow in adolescents, producing extra-gonadal sex hormones. By activating the pituitary-hypothalamus axis, it ushers in adolescence.

Plants contain antioxidants because they undergo oxidative stress. Free radicals also harm plants as the uncoupled oxygen causes cell damage. Free radicals activate nuclear transmission, which destroys CD4 cells and forms a precondition for HIV transmission.

Rasayana therapy is a multidimensional curative treatment which consists of a good diet, regulated lifestyle and supportive family management. It emphasizes the importance of black gram in the diet. *Ghee* plays a very important role as it acts as a solvent for the fat-soluble constituents of the herb. At the molecular level, *rasayana* acts as an anti-inflammatory, oxidative, immunomodulatory agent, and as an antiglycosylation end-product.

Herbal drugs may have a direct antiviral action. They stimulate the body's defence mechanism and reduce its vulnerability to opportunistic infections. Mentha preparations reduce the number of giant cells and have anti-reproductive tract infection activity. *Labiata* has a high content of calcium, magnesium and iron. *Kumari* (*Aloe vera*) tablets (500 mg) contain *asmenon*, which decreases the HIV load. However, no work is being done on this plant in India.

Punica granatum—*funicalac* (*dadima*), *Glycyrrhiza glabra* (*yashtimadhu*) and *Grifula frondosa* have anti-HIV properties. A lot of work is being done on these plants in Japan. *Curcumin* causes transactivation of HIV-1, improves the CD4 count, and decreases apoptosis of CD4 cells and HIV replication.

Bramharasayana contains 50 roots. Roots absorb zinc, magnesium, iron and calcium from the soil, and the diet should be supplemented with those which contain micronutrients. The worship of the *Ficus* tree by women has helped to save it. *Panchavalkala* is obtained from *Ficus* plants, such as *Ficus bengalensis* (*nyagroda*) and *Albizia lebbek* (*sirisha*). Sixty per cent of animals injected intraperitoneally with infective organisms survived when treated with *panchavalkala*, while all the animals in another group not treated with the drug died. *Panchavalkala* is used in drug-resistant osteomyelitis and can cure STDs, but its efficacy in HIV/AIDS is under study. It is used for genital tract infections caused by *Candida* and *Trichomonas vaginalis*. Sperms incubated up to 72 hours with *panchavalkala* and haemeptine showed no change in motility, appearance, etc. while those incubated only with haemeptine died. This demonstrated its safety. Ciprofloxacin-resistant organisms respond to *panchavalkala*. Oral capsules and vaginal pessaries of this drug are in use. The oral capsules are given as chemoprophylaxis before major surgery and drug-resistant osteomyelitis in some major hospitals in Mumbai.

Ayurveda can therefore play a significant role in HIV therapy.

Biospermicides-cum-Microbiocides and HIV/AIDS

G. P. Talwar

Women want a contraceptive which is under their control, and which can be used whenever necessary and not continuously (as with steroids). It should be convenient, effective, safe and, at the same time, save them from sexually transmitted infections, including AIDS. *Neem* is a potent spermicide and could serve as a contraceptive, but its spermicidal property has not been investigated.

Originally, *neem* seeds were used but these were sometimes infected with fungus. Therefore, *neem* leaves were used instead in this preparation. A compound extracted from *neem* leaves is a potent spermicidal agent. UNAIDS brought out a cream with a nanoxine-9 based compound called "Advantages", produced by a company in New York. Though it was supposed to be safe, it caused damage to the vaginal mucosa. While it did kill the organisms causing reproductive tract infections (RTIs), it also facilitated the transmission of AIDS virus by damaging the vaginal mucosa.

The *praneem* polyherbal formulation is a *neem*-based cream or tablet, consisting of three ingredients:

(1) Purified colourless, odourless terpenoid from *neem* (*Azadirachta indica*) (*nimba*) leaves (not very stable if 100% purified);
(2) Saponins from *Sapindus mukoressi* (*arishtaka*) (very stable, more so if pure); and
(3) Mentha citrata oil.

These were standardized on a chromatogram system (PPLC). The three compounds are individually spermicidal and also act synergistically. In combination, their efficacy increases eight- to ten-fold.

Praneem has a wide bactericidal activity on vaginal pathogens and prevents the transmission of HIV/AIDS. Each ingredient, as well as the total formulation, was quality-controlled with respect to the physiochemical profile and biological activity, so that batches of reproductive proportions could be made.

In vitro, it acts on penicillin-resistant *Neisseria gonorrhoeae*, standard urinary tract *Escherichia coli*, as well as multidrug-resistant *E. coli* and the hospital strain of *Staphylococcus aureus*. It also inhibits *Candida albicans*, *tropicalis* and *Candida krusae*. There is good evidence that it acts on the HIV/AIDS virus *in vitro*. Its action on the virus was first tested with the *praneem* pessary.

Praneem was tested *in vivo* by the Pasteur Institute in Paris[1] and at Cornand in Norfolk, USA with excellent results. In the San Diego *in vivo* study, the cream was studied tested at dilutions of up to 50 times. When applied for 6 nights, it killed the HIV-1 virus. *In vivo* studies on the monkey vagina demonstrated that the cream prevented transmission of the virus in the monkey.

Another *in vivo* study was done on mice at the Johns Hopkins University in Baltimore, USA. The mice were infected with the human Herpes simplex virus and Chlamydia after being primed for a week with progesterone. *Praneem* proved to be the most effective antiviral agent among the various preparations tested. It was effective even 8 days later.

Phase I trials (to ascertain its safety) were undertaken in Brazil. There was no adverse local or systemic side-effect. A *praneem* preparation in the form of a tablet was administered for 7 nights. Colposcopy and Papsmear demonstrated that it had no deleterious effect on the vaginal mucosa.

In the Phase II trials (to ascertain efficacy), conducted in Egypt, the live bacterial count (aerobic and anaerobic) in the vagina decreased from 10^{14} to 177,000. Further, the prepration controlled abnormal vaginal discharge.

Phase II trials conducted in Santo Domingo (Dominican Republic) and Salzburg (Austria) yielded excellent results. Two patients with drug resistant balanoposthities were cured by the *praneem* cream. The cream was also seen to control abnormal vaginal discharge in Phase II trials in PGI (Chandigarh). When applied once daily for a week, it clinically cured all vaginal infections. The cream acts as a viricidal agent for HIV/AIDS as well. In Chandigarh, the application of the cream was disliked as the applicator had to be filled with the cream and then applied.

ICMR plans to extend the studies and trials on the antibacterial and viricidal properties of *praneem* in order to obtain further proof of its action.

REFERENCES

1. Talwar G.P., *et al*. Polyherbal formulations with wide spectrum antimicrobial activity against reproductive tract infections and sexually transmitted pathogens. *Am J Reprod Immunol* 2000; 43:144–151.

DISCUSSION

Dr T. Ryan (Oxford)

In the UNAIDS trial in Africa, it was thought that controlling the infection in the vagina and improving barrier resistance and preventing HIV from penetrating would help contain the spread, but the subjects became more susceptible to HIV due to the inflammation and contact dermatitis caused by these antibacterial agents. This subclinical change was seen on biopsy. Since *neem* terpenoids are used they are likely to produce contact dermatitis and vaginal inflammation. Trained persons, such as those available in India, can detect this.

Q. Dr Talwar: Since nonoxyl-9 produced all these complications, we used *neem*—a natural compound. Contact dermatitis should be investigated while developing this formula. Sensitivity tests on the abraded skin of rabbits and accumulated human skin sensitivity tests were conducted for 21 days with the formula.

Q. What happens to the normal cells and useful microorganisms in the vagina?

Ans. Dr Talwar: You mean those which maintain the pH? Not much was done to investigate that aspect.

Comment: *Nimbodichurna* which contains *neem* leaves and bark, was used in Thiruvananthapuram to heal peptic ulcer.

Q. Dr J. Jha: Was it compared to the commonly used allopathic drugs?

Ans. Dr Talwar: At the Postgraduate Institute of Medical Education and Research, the control group was treated with different antimicrobials locally as well as systemically for different conditions. They succeeded in curing the patients. The greatest advantage is that it is a single preparation which can be used for all infections and one need not know the cause of the infection.

Immunomodulation as a Strategy for Restoration of Immunocompetence for Protection Against Opportunistic Infections

Shakti N. Upadhyay

Can immunomodulation be used as a therapeutic strategy for AIDS?

There are two major strategies for fighting a disease. One is chemotherapy, which acts directly against the causative organism and the second is immunomodulation, which entails fortifying the defence mechanisms of the body, but does not act against the organism. The concept of immunomodulation is not new to Ayurveda; rather, it is being rediscovered with modern technology.

In chemotherapy, the strategy is to directly attack the causative organism. It has possible side-effects, such as drug resistance, etc. Immunopotentiation, on the other hand, activates the immune system. Moreover, the immune system can differentiate between normal and abnormal cells. Since immunomodulation does not act directly against the infective agents, there is no question of drug resistance. The effort is to identify the immunomodulatory substances from among natural products.

An antibody can prevent the entry of a virus into a cell, but it cannot act once the virus has entered the cell. It is in this situation that cell-mediated immunity can play a role. The cytotoxic D cells recognize the infected cell and produce factors such as enzymes and various molecules to battle the virus. However, HIV is much more complicated. Since HIV enters the CD cells, the immunomodulatory therapy has to be different from that used for most other infective agents. The therapy must simultaneously kill the virus and boost the immune system. As Ayurvedic drugs attempt to tackle both these factors, they have greater efficacy.

The plants classified as *rasayana* contain a group of compounds which have therapeutic properties and another group which helps in absorption and retention in the system. For this reason, a crude extract would be more effective than a pure extract.

Several studies focusing on macrophages, which produce cytokinins, were conducted. The antimocrobial activity of macrophages can be attributed to nitric oxide. When *Mycobacterium tuberculosis* enters a cell, the macrophages switch off its nitric oxide synthase.

The primary target of the immunomodulatory compounds is believed to be the macrophage, which plays a key role in the generation of an immune response. Macrophages are central to the host's defence mechanism—they not only form the first line of defence against pathogens, but also help generate specific and long-term immunity. They are thus involved in both the afferent and efferent arms of the immune system. In the former, antigen processing and presentation occurs, and in the latter, they function as major effector cells that contain and kill intracellular pathogens. One of the views prevalent among immunologists today is that "a mammalian host unable to activate its macrophages to a state of heightened microbial resistance is susceptible to infection by an intracellular pathogen". Although the phagolysosomal products of macrophages are sufficient to neutralize, degrade and eliminate most foreign bodies, certain infectious pathogens are able to resist this first line of defence and actually thrive within the macrophage, possibly by downregulating the antimicrobial defence mechanisms of macrophages. It appears that host–parasite interactions have evolved in such a way that many parasites have acquired the ability to survive within the host by parasitizing and affecting the immunocompetence of macrophages. The role of macrophages is, therefore, crucial for effective protection against tumours and infections.

Piper longum (*pippali*), a *rasayana* drug which contains piperine, enhances nitric oxide production. In an *in vitro* experiment, cells were lysed 48 hours after being infected and the microbial count was taken. There was no reduction of microbes in the culture. On treatment with different doses of piperine, there was a dose-dependent decrease in the microbial cell count. This matched the amount of nitric oxide produced at the same dose. Further confirmation was provided by the fact that when the nitric oxide synthase inhibitor was added, the killing ability of the macrophages was enhanced. The compound concerned is a molecule from *Piper longum*, which activates macrophages through interaction of cells and then produces nitric oxide, which is responsible for intercellular infection.

The next step was to conduct some *in vivo* studies. However, since there is no animal model for HIV, the researchers had to develop a parallel model, which is not identical to the immunodeficiency produced by HIV infection. As many tumours also cause immunosuppression, a specific tumour cell line was used. This tumour was transplanted and gradually there was a decrease in immunocompetence.

The study demonstrated that there is a reduction in the ability to produce nitric oxide in tumour-bearing animals. Once this was established, the animals were infected with *Mycobacterium smegmatis*, which is a new pathogenic strain that became a fatal infection due to its ability to grow very fast within the animal model and could be the cause of death in this situation.

In another model, the animals were immunocompromised and infected with an opportunistic infection in order to test the *Piper longum* compound. The results obtained were very interesting. The lungs, liver and spleen of the animals infected with *Mycobacterium smegmatis* were examined after a week of infection; homogenization and colony counts were conducted. The colony counts were abnormally high in tumour-bearing animals because nitric oxide production had been blocked, as had the T-cell responses. When the same animals were treated with piperine, almost at the level of control, similar results were obtained. This demonstrates that piperine does not have any direct antimycobacterial effect. Thus, piperine was effective in reducing the microbial cell count when its action was moderated through the immune system, and it did not directly attack the disease-causing agent. This study validates the claim that the plants used in the traditional systems of medicine, especially Ayurveda, could be used as effective co-therapy in the case of HIV also.

Studies were conducted on the effect of *neem* (*Azadirachta indica*) on macrophages from control and treated animals. FITC-coated latex seeds were used to treat the animals with a compound isolated from *neem*. There was a significant increase in their phagocytic activity. Another important criterion for macrophage activation is the expression of mhc class II molecules, which are responsible for the macrophage's antigen-presenting ability. This aspect was investigated by using a specific antibody against them. In the control animals, few cells expressed such molecules, indicative of their antigen-presenting ability. In the animals treated with the immunomodulator, however, there was a significant increase in the number of cells expressing mhc class II molecules indicating that immunocompetence had been enhanced.

A *Leishmania* model was also tested since it involves an intracellular pathogen. These cells are very sensitive to nitric oxide-mediated killing. In the control animals, there was mhc focus in the macrophages but red clots could be seen—these macrophages were the mhc form of surviving *Leishmania*. On the other hand, parasitic clearance was treated with the immunomodulators. *In vivo* studies were conducted on balb/c mice susceptible to *Leishmania* infection. One foot pad was infected and the other served as a control. After a certain degree of inflammation occurred in the wound, the animal was treated with an immunomodulator. This resulted in a significant reduction in the size of the wound. Although there was still some inflammation in some of these animals, it was much less compared to that in the control animals. Again, such drugs do not have any direct anti-*Leishmania* effect, and their therapeutic effect is mediated through the immune system. When such immunomodulators are combined with standard anti-*Leishmania* drugs such as sodium antimonate, the clearance of the parasite is total. Thus, an effective future strategy for therapy is to combine an immunomodulator and an antibiotic or antitumour drug. This probably formed the basis of the Ayurvedic therapeutic strategy, which employs a mixture of various plant materials with different properties.

Another study was conducted to evaluate the therapeutic potential of *neem* compounds on a murine tumour cell line sensitive to nitric oxide-mediated killing. Treatment with these compounds induced regression of subcutaneous P815 tumour implants in DBA/2J mice. The adoptive transfer of macrophages from the treated mice to the tumour-bearing ones also induced tumour regression. This confirmed the macrophage-mediated therapeutic effect of the plant compounds. While the tumours in the control animals became large, those in the treated animals underwent necrosis and became very small. The compounds have no direct antitumor effect, but tumour regression can be induced *in vivo*.

Since *Candida* is one of the major opportunistic infections in HIV cases, immunomodulators which can provide protection against the strain are being screened.

An *in vivo* experiment was conducted in immunocompromised mice which were systematically infected with *Candida*. The kidney was removed and following homogenization, colony counts were undertaken. Even after just one week of treatment, very few colonies could be seen. Continued treatment resulted in a total elimination of *Candida* colonies. This was confirmed by the histopathological analysis.

The traditional system of Ayurveda contains some valuable concepts from which there is a lot to learn. Our results confirm that combining many of these concepts with modern techniques can yield valuable results.

HIV/AIDS and the Use of Condoms

Shashi Kant

What causes AIDS and how to prevent the transmission of the disease is known. That prevention is an effective strategy is also known, as is evidenced by the sustained decline in the incidence of AIDS in Thailand, the continued decrease in its prevalence in Uganda, and the maintenance of low prevalence in Senegal. However, such success has been observed in only a few countries. Globally, the number of cases is still on the rise. This indicates that efforts at prevention are not effective enough. UNAIDS has estimated that 15,000 new infections occur every year.

The four major modes of HIV transmission are:

(1) sexual, mainly heterosexual;
(2) intravenous drug abuse;
(3) blood/blood product transfusion and organ transplant; and
(4) vertical transmission, i.e. from mother to child.

The predominant mode of transmission differs from country to country. As far as Asia is concerned, the epidemic is spreading primarily through heterosexual contact in India, Thailand and Laos, and by intravenous drug abuse in Malaysia, Vietnam and China. Some of the following common interventions/activities may be employed either singly or in combination, to control the epidemic:

(1) Surveillance (sentinel, behavioural, etc.)
(2) Advocacy programmes for human rights
(3) Safe blood supply
(4) Reduction of drug use by reducing the demand/supply
(5) Reduction of the harm entailed in drug use
(6) Programmes to prevent mother-to-child transmission
(7) Voluntary counselling and testing (VCT)
(8) Medical care
(9) Programmes for migrant populations
(10) Health education (life skills)
(11) Treatment and care of sexually transmitted diseases (STDs)
(12) Social marketing of condoms
(13) Programme for 100% condom use

Each of these activities serves at least one of the following objectives of the HIV/AIDS programme:

(1) prevention of infection;
(2) care of people already infected with HIV; and
(3) diminishing the psychological, social and economic impact.

The objectives listed above have inherent merit and constitute a comprehensive response to the epidemic. Since resources are limited, it needs to be determined which of the interventions are the most effective in the prevention of HIV transmission, and how to effectively implement them. The Asian experience indicates that condom promotion (100% condom programme) is the most effective intervention. The moderate-to-less effective interventions are information, education and counselling (IEC) inputs, care of STDs, social marketing of condoms, prevention of needle and syringe exchanges, universal screening of blood donors, medical treatment and VCT. Closure of sex establishments, reduction in drug supply, HIV surveillance and medical treatment of AIDS cases are interventions which cannot be expected to achieve any significant reduction in HIV transmission.

Many men continue to have sexual contact with female commercial sex workers (FCSW) without using condoms. Once infected, they spread the disease to their spouses or other sex partners. An infected spouse may then transmit the infection to her offspring. Studies have shown that more than 90% of HIV-infected women had only one sexual partner, i.e. the husband. The risk of a male client acquiring HIV infection through a single act of unprotected sex with an infected FCSW is estimated to be 0.3% (range 0.01–1.0%). If a condom is used, the risk can be reduced to virtually zero. More than 80% of AIDS patients in India have acquired infection through the heterosexual route. For this reason, the 100% condom programme seems to be the most effective intervention in the Indian context.

There could be two possible strategies for the 100% condom programme:

(1) to supply condoms to the general population and expect them to use these during sexual intercourse with FCSWs; or
(2) to supply condoms to the FCSWs and their clients, and encourage them to use these during sexual intercourse.

The problem with the first approach is that it is logistically very difficult, as well as economically wasteful, and the resultant impact is likely to be low. The second approach is less difficult to implement and very high coverage is achievable. Therefore, it is likely to have a greater impact.

The goal of the 100% condom programme is to prevent heterosexual transmission of HIV among FCSWs and their clients. This is expected to further result in the prevention of HIV transmission among the general population. In order to observe the benefit, it is essential that the condom be used during all sexual contacts (100%) between FCSWs and clients. As commercial sex work is not a recognized occupation in India, there are significant social, political and legal barriers to implementing the programme. The Government of India has recently started implementing targeted interventions among FCSWs through non-governmental organizations (NGOs). Decriminalization and destigmatization of commercial sex work is required for the implementation of the 100% condom programme.

In the government, three sectors are responsible for implementing the programme.

(1) The health sector is responsible for the following activities:
    - STD services
    - Condom supply
    - Providing health education and information to target groups
    - Collecting data on condom use from clients and sex workers with STDs
    - Reporting of non-cooperative sex establishments to the police
(2) Police sector: management of non-cooperative sex establishments
(3) Local administration: coordination between the government sectors and the owners of sex establishments.

The main strategy of the programme is to gain the cooperation of all relevant stakeholders, e.g. the police, healthcare providers, NGOs, brothel owners and gatekeepers, FCSWs and their clients. Efforts should be made to create an environment that enables FCSWs to negotiate on the use of condoms with their clients. If the client refuses to use a condom, FCSW should have the support of brothel owners/gatekeepers to refuse the services. All sex establishments must take measures to deprive the client of services unless he uses a condom.

The key elements in making the programme a success are as follows.

(1) A high level of commitment among all stakeholders
(2) Removal of political, social and legal barriers
(3) Participation of and coordination among all responsible parties
(4) An effective STD programme
(5) An efficient condom promotion programme, as well as logistic management, adequate supply and quality control.

Periodic evaluation of the programme would be required to establish its effectiveness in reducing HIV transmission. The following indicators could be used.

(1) *Incidence of STD.* The programme envisages the existence of an effective STD service which would reduce the prevalence of curable STDs. Many STDs and HIV are transmitted through the sexual route. Therefore, an increase in the incidence of STDs among FCSWs is a good proxy indicator of whether or not condoms are being used during all sexual encounters.

(2) *Prevalence of HIV infection among different target populations.* The programme is expected to reduce the transmission of HIV to the clients of FCSWs. Over a period of time, the prevalence of HIV among the clients should stabilize and then actually start to decline. This indicator could be evaluated through the sentinel surveillance system.

(3) Knowledge, attitudes, behaviour and practices (KABP) surveys on the attitudes and practices relating to condom use among FCSWs and their clients should reveal a positive attitude and an increase in the use of condoms in risky sexual encounters.

(4) The status of implementation of the programme could be ascertained by keeping track of the number of condoms supplied to sex establishments and surveys to determine the percentage of condom use among FCSWs.

The 100% condom programme has already been implemented in Thailand. It has been estimated that from 1989 to 1995, the programme probably prevented over two million cases of HIV infections in the country. The other Asian countries interested in implementing this programme include Cambodia, Myanmar, the Philippines, Viet Nam, China and Indonesia. Needless to say, India would do well to implement such a programme.

An Overview of the Proceedings

G. Bodekar

A journey of a thousand miles begins with a single step. The journey in question refers to the dialogue between HIV/AIDS and traditional medicine, and it does seem like a journey of a thousand miles. The first steps have already been taken and deliberations of the meeting were very significant. The stakes are very high for it involves the health, stability, economic wellbeing and the future of India, and ultimately through India, those of the whole world. The time bomb of HIV/AIDS is ticking, but there is still hope for India if certain known means, public education, and prevention and communication strategies are fully developed. The level of public awareness about the HIV/AIDS crisis is not as high in India as in some African countries. Thailand has been able to turn the tide through conventional means.

India offers more than just the conventional means. The prospect of utilizing the Indian systems of medicine to tackle the crisis provides a source of hope. Steps have already been taken in this direction. Clinicians have been using indigenous systems of medicine to treat HIV/AIDS patients. Many clinics have brought out advertisements, cures and treatments, and the indigenous systems of medicine in the subcontinent have responded wholeheartedly to the crisis. These efforts must be documented and recognized as an informed and sophisticated means of meeting the challenge. The example of Africa is worth emulating. It is the indigenous systems of the African countries that are carrying the burden of clinical cure of AIDS. The ground reality is that people cannot afford antiretroviral therapy. Further, this treatment is not available even for those who can afford it, and most patients cannot afford to go to centres that provide subsidized treatment. Therefore, the affected population remains untreated or avail the traditional forms of treatment, which are affordable and accessible. The same is likely to happen in India. Allopathy cannot ignore this trend. The fact that indigenous systems of medicine are playing an important role, being both available and clinically effective, must be acknowledged. This can be possible only if a process of systematic documentation is initiated.

A beginning can be made by characterizing the potential of indigenous systems, not necessarily through pharmacological but through social research. This would entail an investigation into terms of utilization and epidemiological studies. What is happening has to be captured: (i) the modes of treatment being used by the public; (ii) the options offered by practitioners; (iii) the level of political support being extended across states and by the non-governmental sector; and (d) the institutional response.

On the basis of such information on the consumers, promoters and institutions, a policy and programme can be formulated for the development of indigenous systems. These systems require promotion and support not only in the pharmacological, clinical and molecular aspects, but also from the social point of view.

The most significant feature of the deliberations was the elucidation of the Ayurvedic concepts of disease and health, particularly HIV, before an audience which was not familiar with these concepts. There is both an infectious and a generative basis for HIV development within the Ayurvedic framework. The challenge facing the Ayurvedic fraternity today is to bridge the gap between the traditional and modern systems. There is a need for further conceptualization on *ojas* depletion and the effect of medhas in bioclinical, imunological and ultimately, clinical terms.

Ayurvedic physicians have emphasized the non-infectious genesis of HIV in the past to deny the importance of the role of infection. Using unsubstantiated theories to cling to a false sense of security or giving the people an alibi for denying the sexual basis of HIV, the risk of transmission will only increase. This pitfall should be taken very seriously. The dialogue on the indigenous systems' conceptualization of the disease was extremely valuable and must continue, and scientists should seriously attempt to form links between the different systems. Ayurvedic concepts regarding HIV must be developed, stated and articulated clearly, and should also be published.

Ayurvedic concepts are based on a general framework, but in the context of HIV/AIDS, there is a need develop a guide to clinical practice and evaluation. It has long been argued that research methodologies must be sensitive to indigenous taxonomies. This should be heeded by not only the Ayurvedic fraternity, but the Unani and other schools as well, and their voices should become a part of the dialogue. Siddha proponents, who focus on herbal and mineral cures, must also elucidate and rationalize their principles in terms of clinical potential, methods of action, toxicological assumptions and requirements. Homoeopaths, too, should take part in the dialogue.

The need now is to go beyond this meeting, which dwelt on aspects such as modest clinical reporting, sophisticated clinical evaluation and basic research. The time has come to initiate systematic countrywide research. Once such mapping is completed, it should be presented before a coordination committee, so that the government, funding agencies and research committees can be better informed about the situation and the strengths and lacunae. This would provide a sound basis for a future research agenda and a focused and comprehensive strategy. It would also facilitate coordination of research efforts. Product-oriented research (the technological aspects) and medicine-oriented research would be ideal, as research for the sake of research is an unaffordable luxury in this field. The publication of the deliberations of this meeting will form a landmark document, not just for India but for the entire world. The 8 April issue of *The Lancet* carried a report by Dr Sandra Anderson, a UNAIDS officer in South Africa, who commented on the importance of traditional medicine in combating AIDS in Africa.

This conference has received the support of WHO and UNAIDS would fund the publication of its deliberations. The mainstreaming of this trend is vital if resources are to be mobilized. The traditional sector is beginning to receive a positive response, but this must be recognized and assisted for it to achieve its full potential. Physicians of the traditional systems should ensure that they attain the highest standards within their traditions. They need to not only elucidate the characteristics of the disease, but must also characterize their standards of practice.

Electronic communication in the form of internet and e-mail has brought together the people working against malaria in Africa. The same could be done to tackle HIV/AIDS in India. The dialogue must continue at the local as well as national levels. Research in the various traditional systems should be intra-disciplinary. On the basis of the dialogue, a coordinating committee could prepare a status report on ISM and HIV/AIDS in India, the research currently being done, clinical utilization, promising avenues, currently known cures, and so on. All the relevant institutions and governments should form a partnership and be willing to commit their resources to achieve the task at hand. Political will at the highest level is a serious must. The importance of the huge reservoir of human resources associated with the indigenous systems, as well as the reliance of the majority of India's population on these systems, need to be taken into account. A suitable policy on research and practice will have to be framed. Certain areas of the indigenous sectors are in dire need of investment and training.

The preservation and supply of materials (plants) is just as important as the provision of health services. For example, one of the valuable plants mentioned by Dr Pandey is now a highly endangered and rare species. If plants that offer hope to HIV/AIDS patients become extinct, we have nobody but ourselves to blame. Industries continue to draw upon valuable resources without bothering to renew them. Supply to the natural health sector has been neglected, and it is high time that humans changed their attitude and became responsible custodians of the earth. This brings us to the oft-repeated and relevant question as to what our traditional schools of medicine are doing to promote the local growth of plants (for local use), large-scale plantation, production, forest conservation, and the expansion of forests for the cultivation of important species. It is not only the knowledge imparted by our forefathers that has to be passed on, but also the *Materia medica.*

Policymakers and scientists complain that practitioners of traditional medicine are secretive. However, they have good reason to be so and would not want to share these secrets unless their legitimate rights and economic interests are respected, not only in principle but contractually and legally.

A global conference on traditional medicine and intellectual property rights will be arranged in India in the second half of 2001. India perhaps has more to offer to the world in this regard than any other country. It has successfully overturned the Mississippi patent on turmeric as a wound-healing agent, an achievement which was applauded by the country's traditional medical community. *Neem* is another case in point, besides the CD ROMs being produced on the Indian *Materia medica*, which will be circulated to every patent office in the world. The dissemination of the Indian *Materia medica* no longer depends on the capacity of the investigator to search the databases; it will now be available in every patent office of the world. India is being given full support in showing the way to the other traditional medical communities of the world. The first step in the endeavour to bridge the traditional systems and allopathy has been taken in a spirit if cordiality and the absence of any kind of tension is commendable. Given this spirit, India should be able to successfully share the wealth of knowledge contained in its medical traditions, to attain the highest standards and gain worldwide recognition. India actually has a lot more to offer than what the world thinks possible.

Discussion

Jai P. Narain

The meeting dwelt on two policies that can be used to tackle the HIV/AIDS epidemic. The first policy, which is accepted by most governments, advocates a multisectoral response through the building of partnerships. Undoubtedly, traditional medicine is one of the sectors which could play a very important role, especially in a country like India, considering that it is not only affordable but also culturally acceptable. The HIV/AIDS epidemic has affected almost every part of society and there are already 3.5 million infected people in India. Traditional medicine could provide the care and support these people require so urgently, even at the community level. Further, it would not only prolong their lives, but also improve their quality of life. The second line of attack are antiretroviral drugs. However, as these drugs are extremely expensive, they are not a viable option for countries such as India. We will have to evolve some other system of care, accompanied by voluntary counselling and testing. India's national programme gives priority to the management of opportunistic infections, be it fungal infection, diarrhoea, tuberculosis or even pneumonia, and traditional medicine can certainly play a very important role in this context.

The deliberations of this meeting brought out clearly that there is much positive information with respect to traditional medicine, but scientific evidence is lacking. There is a need to conduct controlled clinical trials to ascertain the benefits in terms of efficacy and toxicity. Traditional medicine can be promoted and advocated only if scientific evidence is collected. The various recommendations of this meeting provide a useful starting point. The areas that require investigation can now be identified and the steps to be taken can be listed. This unprecedented dialogue, in which information and experiences were shared, must now be followed up.

This effort of UNAIDS has evoked interest from WHO. As WHO has identified care and support as one of the core areas, it would certainly be willing to provide whatever technical, or even financial, support is required to further the process that has been initiated.

Homoeopathy Trials in Patients with HIV/AIDS

V.P. Singh

A unique experiment was started in Delhi in 1993 after a few HIV/AIDS cases were referred indirectly by NACO. These patients were suffering from prolonged stress, poor quality of life and lack of nutrition, and also had an inadequate knowledge of a balanced diet.

A book containing information on homoeopathic medicines, as well as methods such as meditation, some exercises, e.g. *suryanamaskar* and *pranayama,* was to be distributed among HIV-infected individuals to help them as many do not have access to physicians.

Homoeopathic physicians have devised a hypothetical model for the treatment of HIV/AIDS. It prescribes a regimen of homoeopathic medicine, psychological counselling, isotonic exercises, sunbathing, *pranayama* and meditation. In addition, it prescribes a supplement of half an ounce of honey and 20–50 g of green lentil sprouts, since HIV-infected patients suffer from a lack of nutrition. Zevit, becosule and multivitamin tablets are also prescribed along with this regimen. The intake of honey is considered compulsory because it is believed that a natural nutritional supplement is assimilated better than synthetic supplements.

Between 1993 and 1998, 39 HIV-infected individuals were covered by this trial. All of them except one haemophilic child, were between 21 and 40 years of age. There were 32 males and 7 females. A lot of time was spent on helping each individual share his/her pain. As far as feedback from the patients was concerned, they were not sure of the efficacy of the medicine but said they felt better when the physician spent time with them. This factor should be taken into account as it indicates that any policy which is formulated should adopt an integrated approach. Apart from recording the clinical benefits, the patient's experience was also recorded. However, there were hardly any laboratory findings.

There was not a single facility for measuring the CD4 cell counts in Delhi in 1993. In 1994, the All India Institute of Medical Sciences (AIIMS) acquired a system, the Facts Scan system, which was not easily accessible to everyone.

Up till now, 10 patients have completed 3 to 7 years in the study. This does not include the new patients who enrolled towards the end of 1998. Two of these ten patients have not gained any weight, but the rest have put on 1 to 8 kg and there has been no exacerbation in their clinical symptoms.

Five of these patients joined the trial between September 1993 and 1994, when facilities to determine CD4 cell counts were not available. In 1999, it was found that their CD4 counts were 281, 390, 412, 341 and 386, respectively. It is significant that even after 9 years of infection (they had all acquired the infection some time in 1991), the CD4 counts should be maintained at 281. This suggests that something in the regimen is stabilizing their immune system. Their health has not deteriorated, they sleep well, have a good appetite and proper bowel movements, and their quality of life is as good as can be hoped for.

According to the CDC (Communicable Disease Centre) classification, a person with a CD4 cell count of 100–200 can be termed an AIDS patient. The count of one of the patients in the trial was 190. Thus, for all practical purposes, he had AIDS and was not expected to survive, but he is still alive. Since he stays far from AIIMS and could not manage to reach in time for blood collection, his CD4 cell count was not taken for years. In December 1998, however, it was found to be 309 and clinically, he is as healthy as any normal person. In the case of other patients, too, the CD4 counts have risen and they are clinically normal. One had a CD4 count of 213 in January 1997 and 385 in August 1999. Another had a CD4 count of 462 in September 1997 and 634 in February 1999. The count of another patient rose from 574 in July 1998 to 760 in October 1999, and that of yet another from 221 in June 1998 to 392 in October 1999. Thus, while the initial regimen may not succeed in enhancing the immune response, it does away with the clinical manifestations and, at the same time, stabilizes the cells responsible for cell-mediated immunity at particular levels.

NACO observed that the first 2000 HIV-infected people monitored in India developed AIDS within 3 to 5 years of contracting the infection, but now it takes 5 to 7 years. Those with infection of 10 years' duration continue to be clinically healthy with a good number of CD4 cells.

Every month, Rs 10,000 has to be spent on two NRTIs and one protease inhibitor. Since this is extremely expensive, most physicians in Delhi prescribe two NRTIs in combination, which costs about Rs 3000. Only about 1% of the affected population in India can afford this. If the Government of India undertakes to treat even one million of the three-and-a-half million HIV-infected people (as reported in 1999), the expenditure would still amount to billions of US dollars, which surpasses India's annual budget. The only way out of this impasse seems to be to take recourse to the 400,000-plus traditional medical practitioners.

For the past 11 years, homoeopaths have been carrying out research on homoeopathic medicines which could provide a promising alternative. The cost of the medicines works out to about Rs 42 per year per patient minus the doctor's fee. If green lentil sprouts and honey are added to the treatment, besides some fruit and vegetables, the cost of treatment would still not exceed Rs 3000 per year.

There is a need for a multiscientific study on all the measures recommended as well as the aspect of psychological support. Plans are afoot to conduct such studies in Chennai, Mumbai and New Delhi, involving homoeopathic physicians, clinicians of modern medicine, microbiologists, immunologists and counsellors. The tasks of laboratory and clinical evaluation should be entrusted to impartial persons not involved in the study. The protocol is being drawn up and will be finalized soon.

The CD4 cell count and viral load remain important parameters for assessing the progression of the disease, as well as the therapeutic effects of the trial. The range of CD4 cell counts among the Indian population would be made public soon. Up till now, assessments are being made according to American or European standards. In India, there are cases of whom only three had CD4 counts of about 500. Those of the rest were between 300 and 400. Moreover, it must be borne in mind that people with a count of about 500 may have all kinds of infections while others with a count as low as 40 may have no clinical manifestation.

A case referred by the National Institute of Communicable Diseases (NICD) had a CD4 count of 40 per mm^3 in January 2000. After 3 months of this therapy, it rose to 202 (the same laboratory, machines, kit and technicians were employed). The medicine given was derived from *Azadirachta indica* (*nimba*). According to a paper presented at the National Institute of Immunology (NII) in 1992 on experiments with *Azadirachta indica*, the extract prepared from the leaves was 60% effective; that from fruits 70% effective; and that from the bark 100% effective against the proliferation of HIV/AIDS. This indicates that a medicine of lower potency contains some molecule of the basic drug which might inhibit the spread of HIV in the blood stream.

When HIV/AIDS infection was first reported in the US, suspicion fell on amyl nitricum/amyl nitrate, which is used by homosexuals. It was only in 1983 that amyl nitricum of 6x potency was defined as an official pharmacopial drug. Homoeopathy is based on the concept that the very substance which causes disease in a healthy person can cure the symptoms and manifestations of the disease. It can be safely assumed that amyl nitricum of 200x potency improves the immune function, as two cases reported definite benefits from such treatment.

Another category of drugs that has proved beneficial is the coded drug, which causes immediate suppression. In the trial, the CD4 counts of the 8 patients who have been taking this drug have risen. Even if repeat tests are carried out on the same day with the same sample, the readings are different. This may be due to factors like the menstrual cycle, anxiety, age and gender. A study would show that on an average, people over 50 years of age have lower CD4 counts, a higher viral load and a greater risk of disease progression than younger persons. The same level will have different implications for a younger person and an older one.

Another study has shown that the viral load is a poor predictor in cases with CD4 counts of less than 50 because the immune system has been devastated. The assessment of viral load is also influenced by the conditions in which the blood is stored, for example, the duration and temperature. There is also always a chance of human error.

Thus, the CD4 count varies with time. Also, if the tests are carried out in different centres, the readings would be different. In view of these variables, margins for these errors have be to allowed for while assessing the therapeutic effects of any drug.

Considering all the factors which have been mentioned, the following suggestions would be useful. Tests are very expensive. Facilities to test the viral load are available only in private laboratories in Delhi. The NICD does not carry out any test and the tests carried out in AIIMS are not readily available. It is suggested that clinical parameters, such as appetite, sleeping pattern, bowel movements and body weight, be included in the protocol. As it is now accepted that the elimination of HIV is not possible, that can be done is to keep the spread under control. This should be the goal, especially in view of the fact that it is possible. For example, the Variola virus, a chickenpox contracted in early childhood, is harboured throughout life without doing much harm. There are other such diseases as well and this factor should be kept in mind while drawing up the protocol.

Note: Patients on amyl nitricum improved within 3 months. Only 6 patients out of 1100 died.

Closing Remarks

Ranjit Roy Chaudhury

The success of this meeting has gone beyond our expectations. We have achieved a lot, and generated a spirit of enthusiasm and real dedication. We must keep up this spirit. On our part, we will do everything that we can. For example, we will try to maintain contact between the participants and keep them together as a body.

I believe that antiretrovirals will become more accessible and less expensive in the near future. A policy has to be framed on which of these drugs we are going to use and which sections of the population we are going to use them on. Are we going to use them on carriers? Probably not. Are we going to use them on those who are developing AIDS? Probably yes. Are we going to use them to prevent mother-to-child transmission? Yes. And for AIDS patients? Probably not. Traditional medicine practitioners will have to be involved in taking these hard decisions. Some of these decisions will have to be taken by the organization which may be formed in the future following this meeting.

We thank all the participants for cooperating with each other. We also thank the speakers, the chairpersons and those who came for the inauguration and provided stimulus to the discussions.

Closing Remarks

V. Ramalingaswami

The dedication and interest shown in tackling the HIV/AIDS epidemic is profound and intense. A great but controversial contemporary figure in the field of physiology, Evan Illich, said: "Every man and woman is a secret teacher, what passes between people, why they talk to each other and what ideas get through, get embedded in the other persons, is not quite known, yet it is obviously an enormous phenomenon that takes place in social life and development is to a large extent dependent on the processes." Even if a vaccine is developed for HIV in 7 years' time, there would still be a need for such secret teaching, messages and communication between people. At this point in time, one can see that the practitioners of traditional Indian systems of medicine are much more effective in general, but there are exceptions. Dr Deivanayagam holds that opportunistic infection should be tackled in accordance with the local ecology and geographical patterns of pathology. The discussion on what the Siddha system of medicine could offer was an eye-opener. Modern medicine and traditional medicine could certainly collaborate in this field. It is synergy, and not disharmony, that is required. In Africa, the indigenous systems of medicine are playing an important role in carrying not only the clinical burden, but also the burden of caring for patients with HIV/AIDS. Africa can teach the world a lot, even in the areas of preventing and reducing the transmission of the disease.

It is a crying shame that the doors of our metropolitan hospitals are often closed to HIV patients. For example, HIV-positive women who go to hospitals for child delivery are often turned away. Modern medicine has to change its attitude towards HIV-positive patients not just in the pursuit of discovering effective and prophylactic agents, but also in the manner treatment is meted out to them. A massive change has to take place within modern medicine. Also, as medicine involves science, hard facts, controversies and denial, new ideas should not be arbitrarily rejected. The true scientific spirit means discussing the idea and proving it to be false upon systematic investigation.

Students of medicine should also be taught about the gentler side of medicine. In tackling HIV, an integrated approach has to be adopted to link all the aspects of the disease—psychological, social, pharmacological, clinical and many others. These deliberations should result in the identification of a goal which emphasizes the need for a continuous process and a synthesis of approaches.

The story of malaria is enlightening. *Quing haotsu* (*artemesin*) was mentioned in the ancient Chinese texts, but this information got buried in the large volume of texts. Thus, years ago somebody had already discovered that there was a particular bark which was very effective against fever with chills. Someone made the connection between chills and fever and malaria. This opened up a new pharmacopoeial world. Years ago, AIDS was recognized in Africa as a "thinning disease". Going back to the community to benefit from whatever help it can offer is the next logical step. We must bring various groups together, publicize the proceedings of this meeting and elicit ideas from the people on how to carry on.

There may be people in the community who are treating HIV/AIDS and perhaps a therapeutic agent could be discovered by investigating what the pundits of the systems of traditional medicine are doing. In the course of such a search, we might also hit upon an agent that modifies the disease or deals with the complications at any level.

The striking thing about this meeting was that it was not a huge one and was held almost anonymously. It was attended by a carefully selected group of people, who agreed to spend two full days demonstrating and presenting their work. Special mention must be made of the scientists from NII, which represents the cutting edge—the immunological edge of science where one would look for an answer to HIV/AIDS.

Many scientists in the US who have changed track to engage in research on HIV have been criticized for doing so for the lure of big money. The finest minds working in all areas of modern science have extended a hand of friendship by agreeing to start on a new journey in the realms of alternative medicine. This meeting which was characterized by genuine goodwill and good, high-quality science, v. as long overdue. Its content was thought out very carefully. It brought together people who have an unquestioned dedication to discovering what the human heritage has to offer, and to try to derive the greatest possible benefit from it.

Intellectual property rights (IPRs) is a topic of tremendous interest and globalization has brought with it a number of problems, which need to be tackled. The meeting was a momentous step, the first of the thousand that need to be taken. The interest, enthusiasm and commitment that was displayed has brought in its wake a feeling of hope and determination to go back and follow up on the issues arising from it. The seeds of development have been sown and each participant, upon return, would try to bring about a change for the better.

Recommendations

M.K. Rajan (New Delhi)

General recommendations
1. Traditional, complementary medicine should be given a status equal to that of modern medicine and not treated merely as an economically affordable system of medicine.
2. The wisdom of traditional health messages, such as those pertaining to diet restrictions (especially in Ayurveda) should be integrated with traditional healthcare.
3. Homoeopathy has been successfully used to treat depression and psychiatric conditions. Its use in the treatment of such conditions amongst HIV/AIDS patients needs to be studied.
4. Ayurvedic medicines which have been used effectively to enhance the stamina, strength, etc. of sports persons need to be studied further in order to document and identify how they can be used to help HIV/AIDS patients.
5. Strengthen community-based cultivation of medicinal plants to prevent their depletion.
6. Develop and implement educational activities to prevent the spread of small epidemics of infection before they become widespread epidemics.
7. Medical students should be exposed to traditional systems of medicine with a view to involving them in the evaluation of traditional medicine at a later point.
8. Explore the possibility of the use of *nimba* (*Azadirachta indica*) and its products in treating HIV/AIDS.
9. Evaluate the services provided by traditional medical practitioners in allopathic hospitals.
10. Document the work done by traditional medical practitioners in the sphere of HIV/AIDS.
11. Continue the dialogue between the practitioners of traditional medicine and modern medicine to arrive at a standardized conceptualization of HIV/AIDS, and develop and implement a coordinated programme which incorporates indigenous treatment to deal with HIV/AIDS.
12. Publish a status report on traditional medicine and HIV/AIDS in India, including all the issues raised at this meeting.
13. Encourage donor agencies to provide full support to traditional medicine.

14. The government should take steps to protect medicinal plants which are fast disappearing due to environmental degradation and uncontrolled use of chemical fertilizers and insecticides.

Research
15. Strengthen the documentation of innovative research in traditional and alternative medicine, and develop national and global networks for the exchange of information.
16. Social research and pharmacological inquiries should precede clinical research.
17. Set up a rapid research response system to support research on the promising aspects of traditional and alternative medicine.
18. Traditional medicine practitioners should establish their own self-regulatory mechanism to establish research priorities and agendas, development agendas, regularize research findings and treatment protocols.
19. Ensure agreements covering intellectual property rights as part of an ethical framework for research.
20. There is a need for a significant increase in funding of research on the impact of traditional medicine on HIV/AIDS.
21. Establish closer linkages between researchers in traditional medicine and financing agencies.
22. Establish a medical advisory council as a central coordinating body comprising all disciplines of medicine, to receive, review and approve research proposals and address other multidisciplinary concerns.
23. Carry out research on research methodology. Map out all research activities carried out in the sphere of traditional medicine in India.

Clinical trials
24. All clinical trials of drugs should include a control group, but not a placebo control group.
25. Conduct a search for and research on more effective Siddha drugs.
26. Combine traditional medicines with antiretroviral therapy in multicentric trials.
27. Set up a multiarm, multicentric control trial using modern drugs, Ayurvedic drugs, homoeopathic drugs, Siddha drugs, etc. to identify the long-term results and the compatibility of these drugs.

Laboratory and testing facilities
28. Establish laboratories for testing the existing as well as new drugs for their immunosuppressive effects.
29. Establish several testing laboratories to carry out viral load assessment as well as measurement of CD4 and CD8 counts, and make these services available to traditional medicine practitioners at affordable costs.

30. Establish an institution along the lines of CDC (Communicable Disease Centre), USA, to which practitioners from all disciplines of medicine can refer technical questions.
31. The ICMR protocol for the cure of HIV infection/AIDS needs to be revised with inputs from medical practitioners from all disciplines.

Dr C.N. Deivanayagam (Chennai)

Medical Advisory Council or Health Advisory Committee
A non-governmental registered society should be set up, which will advise the government and the community on every aspect of health and disease.

1. It will help formulate guidelines on areas of priority in the health sector and in disease research, now done by the Scientific Advisory Committee.
2. It will help promote Indian systems of healthcare through the growth of the resources required for the drugs used by them.
3. It will draw up guidelines for daily exercise regimens, the quality of air that we (Au ??) breathe and its availability, the quality of potable water, and the promotion of natural and nutritious food.
4. It will function as a prompt clearinghouse with regard to the need, viability and urgency of any research proposal forwarded in India or abroad.
5. It will advise the State and Central Governments on short and long-term plans for the promotion of health and reduction of disability.
6. It will advise the education and social sectors, both non-governmental and governmental, on the content of health education in the school curriculum and promote healthy living through schools. A possible suggestion could be the inclusion of physical training singing or dancing lessons in school.
7. When any problem is referred to this body, it will help formulate integrated approaches to the traditional Indian systems of medicine and modern biomedical systems.
8. It will help provide guidelines for documentation and publication. This body will be a non-governmental registered society. It will be more in the nature of a health advisory body or think tank which includes traditional medical practitioners, advisors, NGOs and non-medical people.

Dr Lalit M. Nath (WHO, New Delhi)—Additional recommendations

1. NACO should initiate a skill-building and training process for programmes advocating the use of condoms. Such training should cover the health providers of all systems of medicine.

2. Basic counselling and skill-building programmes should be initiated for practitioners of all systems of medicine.
3. Identify a panel of epidemiologists/clinical experts who can be used as consultants while designing or redefining projects throughout the country, and who would be available to practitioners of the various systems of medicine.

Dr R. Kuttan (Thrissur, Kerala)

Since many plants and formulations were mentioned and discussed in this meeting, a uniform formulation could be arrived at with the help of traditional practitioners. Strict standards should be maintained while preparing the formula, which could then be tested. This would lend uniformity to the whole process. One could then proceed to hold multicentric clinical trials of the formula.

Dr Vasantha Muthuswamy (ICMR, New Delhi)

The recommendations arising from this meeting should be clear-cut to facilitate follow up. The responsibility should be given to a certain individual or organization, otherwise everything will remain only on paper. What we need is an all-India coordination committee to coordinate the developments in the different systems of medicine. Such a body would serve as a common platform for discussing the results, arriving at decisions and responding to the recommendations. These tasks should be taken up immediately so that clinical trials can be held to provide evidence for our claims. The responsibility of setting up this an all-India coordination committee should be given to the ISM.

The suggestion to set up a non-governmental committee is valid, but it will take time for such a body to become fully functional. The immediate need is for all-India coordinating committee involving all systems of medicine. We know that definite leads have been provided by the alternative systems of medicine. Large multicentric clinical trials are required to follow up these leads. This responsibility can be given to ICMR, whose protocol has been followed by everybody. As the protocol was developed a few years ago, it needs some alterations in view of the latest ethical guidelines being followed worldwide. Since the practitioners of different systems are going to undertake clinical trails, they need to be trained in the methodology of clinical trials for these trials to be globally acceptable.

An inventory should be made of the available treatment modalities. Perhaps separate inventories will have to be made under each system. For the time being, the inventory should cover whatever positive leads are available. We are aware of our responsibility to further the process that has been started and the next such conference will reveal whatever progress has been made.

Jai P. Narain (WHO, New Delhi)

Anybody who wants any information should be able to get it from a "clearinghouse" by writing.

Clear-cut recommendations on matters pertaining to the generation of scientific evidence through controlled clinical trials should be written out explicitly. The roles to be played by different agencies, such as NACO, ICMR and WHO, should also be identified. The government should bring out some guidelines on advertisements inserted in the newspapers by those claiming to have cures, as many of these are misleading.

Sanskrit terms used in the text

Anuloma and pratiloma
Artha
Ashtadhatu
Ashtamaithun
Asthanedamaithun
Atma
Brahmacharya
Chaturvedapurushartha dharma
Dharak
Dharmavithebhisu kamoshi bharth shava
Dhatukshinata
Doshas
Jeevaneeya agumardhaka
Jeevaniyo
Kama
Keli, urikshnam, bhuyabhasnam, sankalp, adhyasaystha
Moksh
Ojas
Ojasksaya
Pachaniyum

Panchakarma
Panchamahabhoot
Pathya
Prasantmaindrayana
Pratiloma rajayakshama
Rajamriyanka
Rasadhatukshaya
Rasayana
Roga vinischaya
Samarprapati
Sandaxpani
Sankramak rogas
Sannipataka jwar
Santarpak
Saptadhatu
Satvarardhaka dravyas
Shukradhatukshaya
Sitophaladi churan
Swarnpanpati
Vasantamalti
Vijayams

List of Contributors

1. Dr. G. Bodeker, Chairman, Global Initiative for Traditional Systems of Health, Green College, University of Oxford, Oxford, U.K.
2. Vaidya Suresh Chaturvedi, Ayurvedic Consultant, Ville Parle, Mumbai.
3. Dr. S.A. Dahanukar*, Professor & Head, Deptt. of Pharmacology & Therapeutics, Seth G.S. Medical College & KEM Hospital, Parel, Mumbai.
4. Dr. C.N. Deivanayagam**, Medical Superintendent, Government Hospital for Thoracic Medicine, Chennai.
5. Dr. Shashi Kant, National Consultant, Office of WHO Representative to India, New Delhi.
6. Dr. R. Kuttan, Research Director, Amala Ayurvedic Hospital, Kerala.
7. Dr. Jai P. Narain, Regional Advisor, WHO-SEARO, New Delhi.
8. Dr. H.S. Palep, Honorary Professor Obstetrics & Gynaecology, Grant Medical College, Mumbai.
9. Dr. V.N. Pandey, National Consultant – Indian Systems of Medicine, Ministry of Health & Family Welfare, New Delhi.
10. Mr. M.K. Rajan, Delhi Society for Promotion of Rational Use of Drugs, National Institute of Immunology, Aruna Asaf Ali Marg, New Delhi.
11. Professor V. Ràmalingaswami, National Research Professor, New Delhi.
12. Dr. S. Rohatgi, Chairman, Hind Chemicals Limited, Kanpur.
13. Professor Ranjit Roy Chaudhury, President, Delhi Society for Promotion of Rational Use of Drugs, New Delhi.
14. Dr. Q.B. Saxena, Deputy Director General, Indian Council of Medical Research, New Delhi.
15. Vaidya Shriram Sharma, President, Mittal Ayurvedic College, Mumbai.
16. Dr. V.P. Singh, Assistant Director & Programme Officer (HIV/AIDS), Central Council for Research in Homoeopathy, New Delhi.
17. Dr. G.P. Talwar, Director Research & Principal Trustee, Talwar Research Foundation, New Delhi.
18. Dr. Shakti Upadhyay***, Scientist, National Institute of Immunology, New Delhi.

---

*Present Address: Dean, BYL Nair Ch. Hospital & TN Medical College, Mumbai.
** Present Address: President, Health India Foundation, Chennai.
*** Present Address: Research Director, Reliance Life Sciences, Mumbai.